V. Hach-Wunderle · P.P. Nawroth (Eds.)

Life-Threatening Coagulation Disorders in Critical Care Medicine

Springer
Berlin
Heidelberg
New York
Barcelona
Budapest
Hong Kong
London
Milan
Paris
Santa Clara
Singapore
Tokyo

V. Hach-Wunderle · P.P. Nawroth (Eds.)

Life-Threatening Coagulation Disorders in Critical Care Medicine

Translated by T.C. Telger

With 19 Figures and 4 Tables

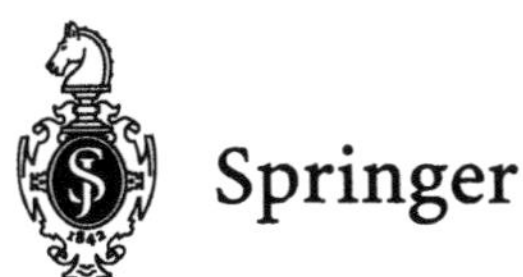 Springer

Priv.-Doz. Dr. med. VIOLA HACH-WUNDERLE
William-Harvey-Klinik, Abt. für Innere Medizin
Am Kaiserberg 6
61231 Bad Nauheim
Germany

Priv.-Doz. Dr. med. PETER P. NAWROTH
Medizinische Klinik I, Universität Heidelberg
Bergheimer Straße 58
69115 Heidelberg
Germany

ISBN-13:978-3-540-61475-3   e-ISBN-13:978-3-642-60490-4
DOI: 10.1007/978-3-642-60490-4

Library of Congress Cataloging-in-Publication Data. Lebensbedrohliche Gerinnungsstorun-
gen in der Intensivmedizin. English. Life-threatening coagulation disorders in critical care
medicine/V. Hach-Wunderle. P.P. Nawroth, eds.: translated by T.C. Telger. p. cm.
Includes bibliographical references and index.ISBN-13:978-3-540-61475-3 (softcover:alk. paper)
1.Disseminated intravascular coagulation. 2.Cardiovascular emergencies. I. Hach-Wunderle,
V. (Viola) II. Nawroth, P.P. (Peter P.). 1954-   . III. Title. [DNLM: 1. Disseminated
Intravascular Coagulation. 2. Postoperative Hemorrhage – prevention & control. 3. Critical
Care – methods. WH 322 L722 1997a] R6647.D5L4313 – 1997 616.1'57 – dc20 DNLM/DLC for
Library of Congress 97-29356

Cover design: Design & Production GmbH, Heidelberg

Typesetting: Scientific Publishing Services (P) Ltd, Madras

The text printed in this book was taken directly from data supplied by the editors.

SPIN: 10539475   23/3134/SPS – 5 4 3 2 1 0 – Printed on acid-free paper

Preface

Hypercoagulability and bleeding are problems physicians frequently encounter when treating intensive care patients. The coagulation mechanism is a tightly controlled system. Its balance is disturbed in conditions such as septicemia, trauma, shock, and others. The disturbances may be local or disseminated and the therapeutic options available are limited and nonspecific: limited since in most circumstances they may not affect the underlying disease and are similarly independent of the pathogenic mechanism; nonspecific since they cannot be specifically targeted to the problem of local or systemic disturbance of coagulation. Furthermore, increased and decreased coagulability may be present at the same time. Activation of coagulation may lead to fibrin deposition and decreased hemostatic capacity, as seen in disseminated intravascular coagulation.

New diagnostic approaches for acquired disorders of coagulation have been developed and form a new basis for therapeutic strategies. Despite this progress, many physicians are aware of the problem that, especially for intensive care patients, a treatment very often has to be selected before diagnostic procedures can be completed. We also know that for many diseases rare occurrence or the heterogenity of the patient population make it quite difficult to conduct clinical studies which prove that a therapeutic regimen is efficacious. Thus, much discussion about coagulation disorders in critically ill patients is still necessary. Even so, it is important to provide guidelines for handling these problems.

This book aims to inform the reader about the current status of the discussion, but at the same time offer a basis for making bedside decisions, where discussions are sometimes important, but which cannot replace good medical practice.

Bad Nauheim/Heidelberg,
September 1996

VIOLA HACH-WUNDERLE
PETER P. NAWROTH

Contents

List of Contributors

H. BÖHRER, M.D.
  Department of Anesthesiology, University of Heidelberg,
  Im Neuenheimer Feld 110, 69120 Heidelberg, Germany

A. GREINACHER, M.D., Ph.D.
  Department of Immunology and Transfusion Medicine,
  Ernst Moritz Arndt University,
  Sauerbruchstrasse, 17487 Greifswald, Germany

M. KÖHLER, M.D., Ph.D.
  Department of Transfusion Medicine,
  Georg August University Medical Center,
  37070 Göttingen, Germany

P.P. NAWROTH, M.D.
  Medical Clinic I, University of Heidelberg,
  Bergheimer Strasse 58, 69115 Heidelberg, Germany

B. PÖTZSCH, M.D., Ph.D.
  Department of Hemostasis and Transfusion Medicine,
  Kerckhoff Hospital,
  Sprudelhof 11, 61231 Bad Nauheim, Germany

H. RIESS, M.D., Ph.D.
  Department of Internal Medicine,
  Virchow Medical Center, Humboldt University,
  Augustenburger Platz 1, 13353 Berlin, Germany

I. SCHARRER, M.D., Ph.D.
  Center of Internal Medicine,
  J.W. Goethe University,
  Theodor-Stern-Kai 7, 60596 Frankfurt am Main, Germany

R. SCHERER, M.D.
  Department of Anesthesiology,
  Essen University Medical Center,
  Hufelandstrasse 55, 45122 Essen, Germany

Part I

Disseminated
Intravascular Coagulation (DIC)

CHAPTER 1

Pathophysiology, Presentation, and Treatment of Conditions Associated with DIC

H. Böhrer and P.P. Nawroth

Summary

Disseminated intravascular coagulation (DIC) is a complex process from both the diagnostic and therapeutic standpoint. There are a number of underlying disorders that can trigger DIC. Its clinical manifestations are diverse, its diagnostic criteria have not been uniformly defined, and various therapeutic strategies, some still experimental, have been advocated for patient use. Since morbidity and survival depend mainly on the specific cause of the DIC, and because prospective, randomized multicenter studies have not done to verify treatment efficacies, general treatment guidelines for DIC cannot be formulated.

DIC is not a separate disease entity but occurs as a sequela or complication of a severe underlying disorder. The activation of blood coagulation in the setting of these disorders induces excessive intravascular clotting that can be manifested in various ways. First, there is widespread generation and deposition of fibrin, leading to microthrombus formation in multiple organ systems. Second, the persistent widespread activation of the coagulation system leads to the consumption of clotting factors. This process is intensified by impaired hepatic synthetic function and a shortened half-life of clotting factors due to proteinase activation. Because of this consumption and the resultant thrombocytopenia, microthrombosis in DIC may be complicated by severe hemorrhagic complications.

Underlying disorders that may be associated with DIC in critically ill patients	
	• Sepsis
	• Shock
	• Multiple injuries
	• ARDS
	• Hemolysis
	• Graft rejection
	• Obstetric complications
	• Poisonings
	• Pancreatitis
	• Snakebite
	• Malaria
	• Leukemias

Sepsis

Sepsis is considered the leading cause of acute DIC [44]. DIC is among the most frequent complications of sepsis, which is almost invariably associated with coagulation abnormalities [23]. Patients in septic shock who develop DIC have a higher mortality rate than patients who do not manifest DIC [67]. DIC, with its ubiquitous microthrombosis, plays a key role in the pathogenesis of organ dysfunction in septic shock, and DIC may be considered a major factor in the development of multiple organ failure.

In recent years efforts have been made to define or redefine sepsis as a pathologic condition [13, 27, 203]. Prompted by the observation that a microbial trigger cannot be identified in many patients who have clinical manifestations of sepsis, Bone [27] and his colleagues differentiated the symptom complex into sepsis, septic syndrome, and septic shock. In Europe, Vincent [205] and his group classified septic states into bacteremia, septicemia, and sepsis. From these discussions has emerged the concept of the systemic inflammatory response syndrome (SIRS) (Fig. 1, [24]), which holds that sepsis may be present even though a pathogen is not detectable upon examination. The hallmark of this syndrome is a systemic inflammatory response to infection, surgery, burn, pancreatitis, or trauma. The systemic response of the organism to these triggers can range in severity from a relatively mild reaction to septic shock.

Clinical Manifestations of Sepsis

The clinical features of sepsis include:

1. Core temperature > 38.5°C, with hypothermia (< 35.5°C) occurring in 1%–10% of patients [6].
2. Tachycardia.
3. Tachypnea, which may present initially as hyperventilation with respiratory alkalosis.
4. Abnormal WBC (see below). Leukocytosis is generally present, but a few patients may exhibit leukopenia.

General laboratory manifestations of sepsis

- **Blood count:**
  - Leukocytosis > 15 000/mm^3 or leukopenia < 3500/mm^3
  - Left shift, toxic granulation

- **Changes in the coagulation system:**
  - Fall in platelet count > 30%/24 h
  - Decrease in antithrombin III

- **Metabolic abnormalities:**
  - Hyperlactatemia
  - Hyperglycemia
  - Hypophosphatemia

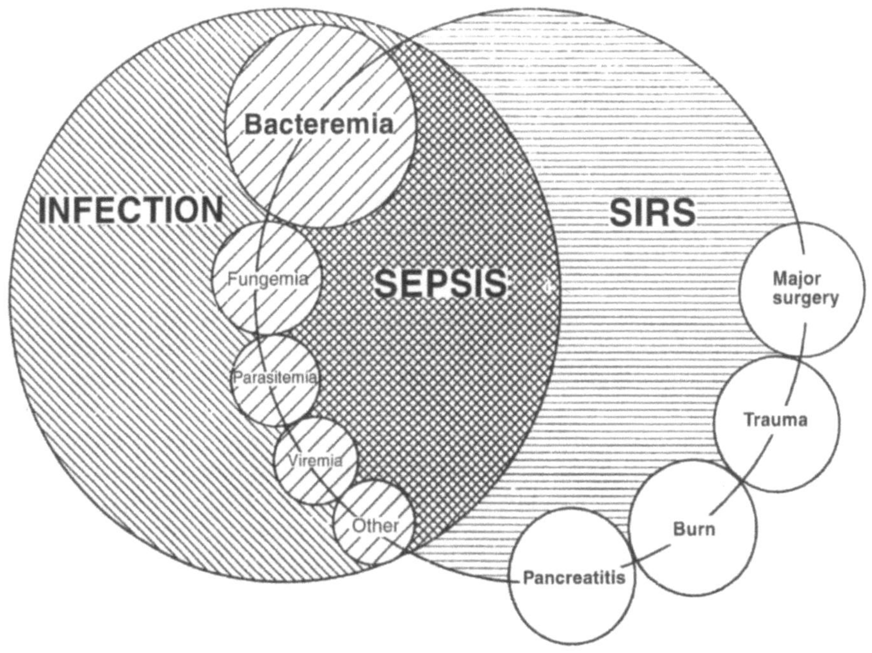

Fig. 1. Relationship between systemic inflammatory response syndrome (SIRS), sepsis, and infection (modified from [3])

Further symptoms can result from changes in organ perfusion:

- Central nervous system: acute confusion and unrest [21].
- Lung: respiratory insufficiency.
- Kidney: oliguria or anuria with increased solute retention.
- Circulation: hypotension with systemic systolic pressures < 90 mm Hg or a fall in blood pressure > 40 mm Hg. In patients with fully established septic shock, the hypotension tends to persist despite volume replacement or treatment with inotropic agents.
- Disturbance of coagulation and fibrinolysis ranging to the complete picture of DIC.
- Complement system activation.

Laboratory abnormalities that may be associated with gram-negative sepsis are listed in Table 1. The course and prognosis of sepsis depend in part on the

Table 1. Potential laboratory signs of gram-negative sepsis

	Prevalence (%)
Positive blood cultures	10–45
Demonstration of endotoxin	60
Thrombocytopenia < 100 000/mm^3	10
More than 30% fall in platelet count	80
Antithrombin III < 70% of normal	80

underlying disease. Fulminant forms of sepsis are especially likely to occur in immunosuppressed patients. Worldwide data indicate a 40%–60% mortality rate for septic shock. The mortality figures are lower for shock due to sepsis resulting from lower urinary tract disease. The concomitant presence of hypothermia implies a significant increase in mortality [43]. Septic shock in patients with hepatic cirrhosis is invariably fatal [137].

With septic shock that is refractory to treatment, individual organs such as the lung, kidney, and liver start to fail within 1–3 days. Unless the vicious cycle is interrupted, multiple organ system failure is inevitable [160], and death is almost certain to occur.

Scoring systems are commonly used in assessing the condition and prognosis of intensive care patients [145]. While the APACHE score is widely used for the general assessment of ICU patients [108], special grading systems are used for septic patients. The septic scoring systems most commonly used in recent years were introduced by Elebute [58] and Stevens [185] in 1983; these systems assign higher scores as the severity of the sepsis increases (see Table 2). Baumgartner [11] recently published a newer method for grading the severity of septic shock. Sepsis scores are used not only for assessing prognosis [54] but also as a guide for selecting specific therapeutic interventions [55].

Pathophysiology

Endotoxin, Cytokines

One of the most potent triggers of DIC is bacterial coat lipopolysaccharide (LPS), or endotoxin, which occurs in the membrane of gram-negative bacteria. Endotoxin is composed of three regions: an O-specific side chain, a core polysaccharide, and a lipid A region that is virtually identical in all gram-negative species [74]. In a 1988 study by Michie [113], maximum plasma levels of tumor necrosis factor (TNF) were measured in 13 volunteers 60–90 min after the intravenous injection of endotoxin. This factor is of major importance, functioning as a central mediator of sepsis [196]. The interleukin-1 concentration rises shortly after the maximal release of TNF, reflecting the role of interleukin-1 as a second primary mediator. The rise in these proinflammatory cytokines is followed by an elevation of interleukin 6, one action of which is to initiate the synthesis of acute phase proteins in the liver [49]. Efforts in recent years to correlate the plasma levels of cytokines with clinical outcomes have shown that the initial levels of interleukin 6 are a useful prognostic indicator, with higher levels of interleukin 6 implying a less favorable prognosis [39, 143].

The mechanisms of cytokine release in sepsis have been studied more closely in recent years. LPS binds to lipopolysaccharide-binding protein (LBP, [167]), and the LPS–LBP complex interacts with the CD14 receptor on macrophages [212], inducing the release of cytokines by the macrophage (Fig. 2). This initiates a cascade of various mediator systems (Fig. 3) that alter the levels of bradykinin, histamine, eicosanoids (prostaglandins, leukotrienes, throm-

Table 2. System for grading the severity of surgery-related sepsis. The scores for local effects, body temperature, secondary effects, and laboratory data are added together. In this way a specific numerical value can be assigned to the patient's septic state. (After [58])

	Score
1. Scoring of local effects	
Wound infection requiring	
Dressing change once daily	2
Dressing change more than once daily	4
Peritonitis	
Localized	2
Generalized	6
Chest infection	
Clinical or radiologic signs without a productive cough	2
Clinical or radiologic signs with a productive cough	4
Full clinical picture of lobar or bronchopneumonia	6
Deep-seated infection (e.g., subphrenic abscess, 6 osteomyelitis)	
2. Scoring of body temperature	
Maximum daily temperature (°C)	
36–37.4	0
37.5–38.4	1
38.5–39	2
> 39	3
< 36	3
Minimum daily temperature > 37.5°C	1
Two or more temperature peaks > 38.4°C in one day	1
3. Scoring of secondary effects	
Jaundice (in the absence of preexisting hepatic disease)	2
Metabolic acidosis	
Compensated	1
Uncompensated	2
Renal failure	3
Neurologic impairment (confusion, etc.)	3
Bleeding diathesis in setting of DIC	3
4. Scoring of laboratory data	
Blood culture	
Single positive culture	1
Two or more positive cultures 24 h apart	3
Single positive culture with history of invasive surgery	3
Single positive culture + cardiac murmur and/or splenomegaly	3
Leukocyte count	
12 000–30 000/mm^3	1
> 30 000/mm^3	2
< 2500/mm^3	3
Hemoglobin level	
7–10 g/dl	1
< 7 g/dl	2
Platelet count	
100 000–150 000/mm^3	1
< 100 000/mm^3	2
Plasma albumin level	
31–35 g/l	1
25–30 g/l	2
< 25 g/l	3
Total bilirubin in the absence of jaundice > 1.5 mg/dl	1

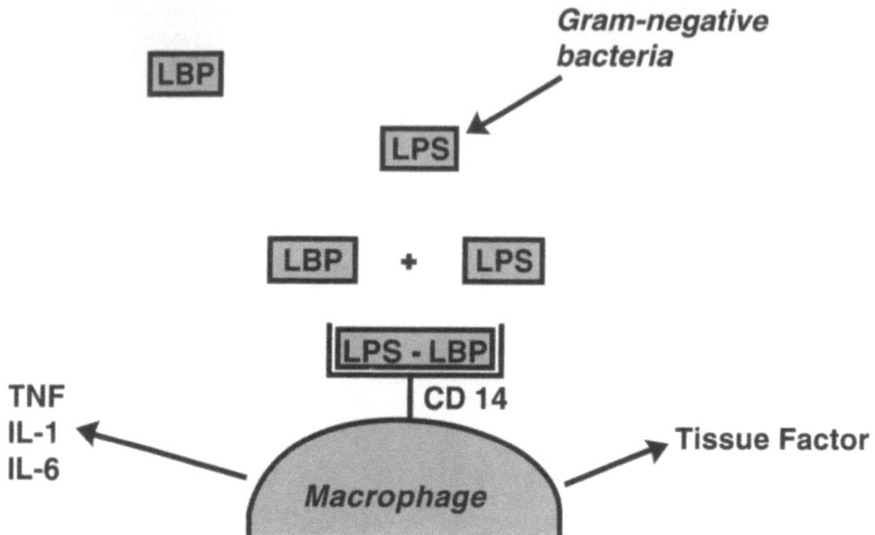

Fig. 2. Endotoxin (*LPS*) forms a complex with lipopolysaccharide-binding protein (*LBP*) that induces cytokine release after binding to the CD_{14} receptor

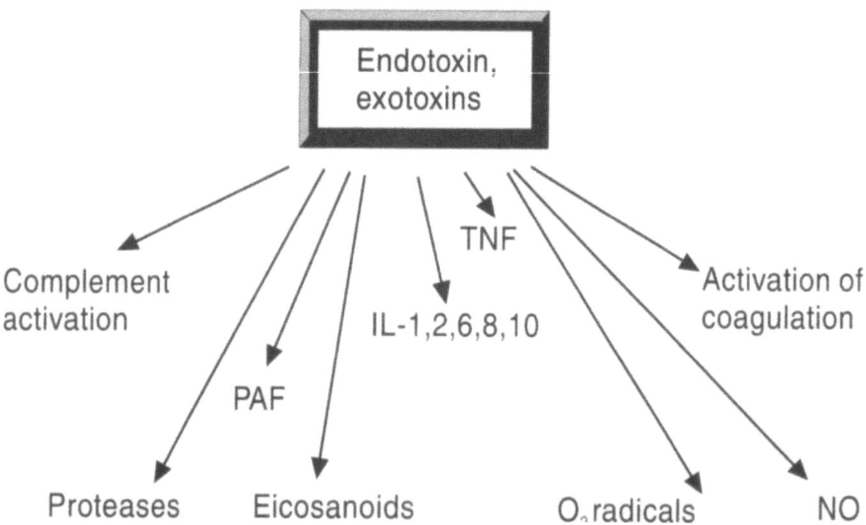

Fig. 3. Endotoxin and exotoxin release in sepsis leads to "flooding" of the organism with a variety of mediators. *TNF,* tumor necrosis factor; *IL,* interleukin; *PAF,* platelet-activating factor

boxanes, prostacyclin), complement fractions, oxygen radicals [107], platelet activating factor [4], and clotting factors, culminating in the development of a general endothelial inflammation. The resulting overall septic state with incipient organ failure have been termed "autotoxic horror" in the recent literature [10].

Leukocyte-Endothelial Interactions

Neutrophilic granulocytes play a key role in the pathogenesis of inflammatory tissue injury [210]. Inflammatory processes start at the microcirculatory level with an increase in granulocyte "sticking." This increased adherence of circulating granulocytes to the vascular endothelium enables the granulocytes to exert their destructive effects on the vessel wall. Their adherence is controlled by the expression of adhesion molecules on the cell surface.

Unstimulated granulocytes show a low surface density of these adhesion molecules. When stimulated, the granulocytes express various glycoproteins on their outer cell membrane, collectively termed the CD_{11}/CD_{18} complex [182]. Meanwhile the stimulation of endothelial cells induces the expression of adhesion molecules on the endothelial cell surface. These endothelial adhesion molecules include endothelial leukocyte adhesion molecules (ELAMs, E-selectin), intercellular adhesion molecules (ICAMs), and vascular cell adhesion molecules (VCAMs). The interaction of the adhesion-mediating endothelial and leukocytic glycoproteins initiate the coupling of humoral to cellular mediator systems.

Disseminated Intravascular Inflammation

A number of other phenomena that take place in the intravascular compartment can induce the activation of leukocytes. One possible cause besides bacteria and their products is mechanical traumatization of the blood due to cell saving (Fig. 4) or other mechanisms. This leukocyte activation syndrome incites a widespread intravascular inflammatory response known as "disseminated intravascular inflammation" (DII) [35].

Capillary Leakage

The systemic inflammatory response that occurs in sepsis leads to capillary leakage. Acute pulmonary failure, for example, starts with an increase in the permeability of the pulmonary capillary endothelium (Fig. 5). The endothelial disruption allows inflammatory fluid and cells to shift from the intravascular compartment into the pulmonary interstitium and finally into the alveolar spaces. This leads to alveolar engorgement, the inactivation of surfactant, and alveolar collapse, resulting in a ventilation-perfusion mismatch with hypoxemia and diffuse pulmonary infiltrates. Analogous impairment of capillary permeability occurs in other organ systems, leading to organ dysfunction.

The proinflammatory cytokines TNF and interleukin 1 increase the permeability of the endothelial cells [36, 159] in a process that may involve a "vascular permeability factor" [42]. This increased permeability is manifested approximately 6 h after it is triggered and becomes maximal in 12–24 h as the combination of cytokines exert potentiating effects. Platelet-activating factor also increases vascular permeability [110, 180] as it interacts synergistically

Fig. 4

Monocytes and granulocytes in cell saver blood
Plasma
Cells
Leukocyte rolling
Platelet-leukocyte deposition
Activated granulocytes and monocytes

Fig. 5
▼

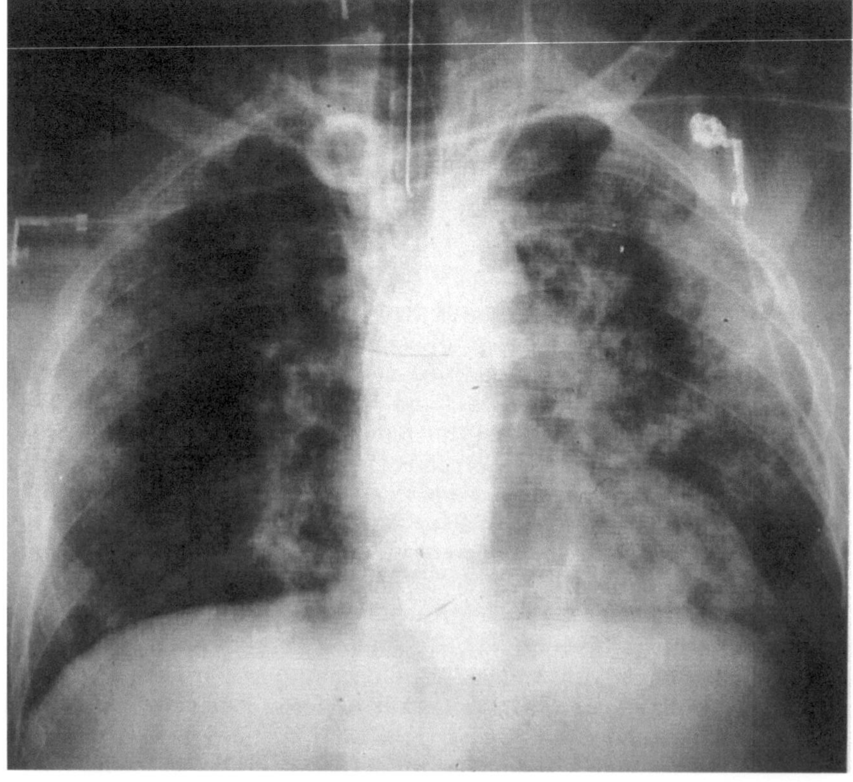

with various cytokines. The shift of fluids and proteins can be demonstrated experimentally with the use of radiolabeled proteins such as transferrin, and the local uptake of radioactivity can be quantitated by scintigraphy [169]. Capillary leakage is manifested clinically by a deterioration of respiratory or ventilatory parameters and by general fluid retention, which may be apparent on the back of the hand (see Fig. 6).

Ischemia reperfusion is consistently associated with capillary leakage. Ischemia reperfusion involving the heart, bowel, liver, or lower extremities not only causes local reperfusion injury but can induce similar phenomena in other organs such as the lung, giving rise to the term "remote microvascular injury." The ischemia-reperfusion process activates neutrophils, monocytes, and macrophages leading to the release of oxygen-derived free radicals, eicosanoids, cytokines, and activated complement production. The resulting changes in endothelial cell function lead to altered permeability with capillary leakage. Such phenomena are known to occur in shock, after prolonged cardiopulmonary bypass, and in association with acute, major vascular surgical procedures.

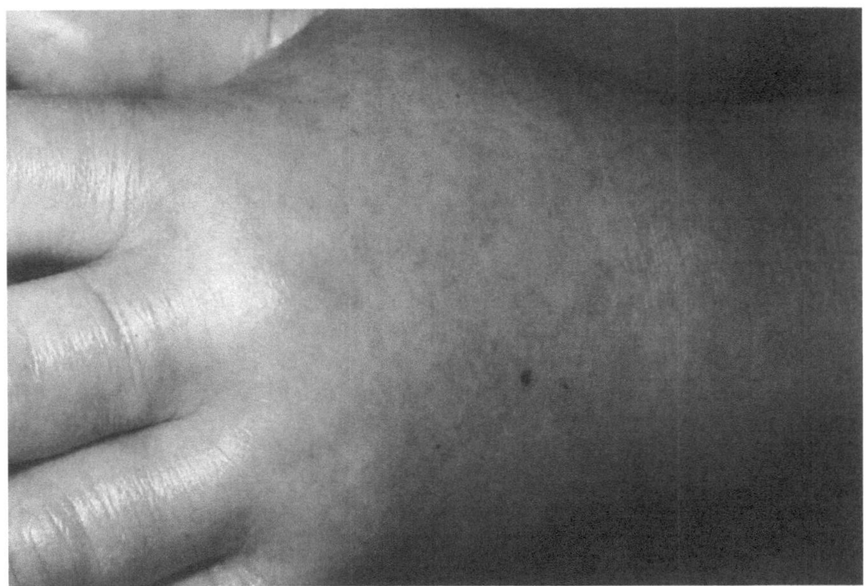

Fig. 6. Dorsal hand edema in a patient with capillary leakage

Fig. 4. Mechanism of leukocyte activation by cell saving. A leukocyte activation syndrome develops which Bull et al. termed "disseminated intravascular inflammation" (DII) [35]

Fig. 5. Typical cloudy infiltrates caused by pulmonary capillary leakage

Activation of Coagulation

The elevation of circulating cytokine levels is followed by a significant rise in the markers for thrombin generation (prothrombin fragments F_1 and F_2, thrombin–antithrombin complex) and markers for the conversion of fibrinogen to fibrin (fibrinopeptide A, fibrin monomers, [201]). A similar activation of the coagulation system can be observed by injecting subjects with TNF [199]. The concurrent administration of pentoxifylline and endotoxin in chimpanzees blocks the endotoxin-induced expression of TNF, with an associated inhibition of clotting activity [115]. Thus, TNF is not only a central mediator in the cytokine cascade but also represents a critical mediator of endotoxin-induced procoagulant activation.

Thrombin generation can occur via the intrinsic or extrinsic pathway. Initial studies showed very low levels of Hageman factor (factor XII) in septic patients [128], with the Hageman factor in the intrinsic system playing an essential role. Also, in vitro studies showed that high concentrations of endotoxin can directly activate the Hageman factor [105]. It was formerly concluded from these studies that the intrinsic system was responsible for the activation of coagulation.

More recent studies have shown, however, that the extrinsic pathway is chiefly responsible for initial activation of the coagulation system in sepsis, making this a tissue-factor-dependent process (see Fig. 7, [38]). The injection of endotoxin or TNF in experimental subjects is followed by marked, factor X-mediated thrombin formation with no significant change in markers for activation of the intrinsic system such as factor XII-C1 inhibitor complex, kallikrein-C1 inhibitor complex, or factor IX activation peptide. Marked expression of tissue factor was observed in primates following the infusion of lethal doses of *Escherichia coli* [56]. Also, in vivo studies have shown that endotoxin, TNF, and interleukin 1 induce tissue-factor expression on monocytes and endothelial cells [34, 57, 106, 130]. Tissue factor binds factor VIIa, forming a tissue factor-factor VIIa complex that is responsible for the conversion of factor X to factor Xa. Clinical studies also have demonstrated an increase in tissue-factor expression on monocytes in children with meningococcal sepsis [141]. Further evidence for the dominant role of the extrinsic system in this activation process comes from studies in chimpanzees with experimental bacteremia or endotoxemia in which tissue factor or factor VIIa was blocked with monoclonal antibodies [15, 115, 192]. Endotoxin-induced thrombin formation and fibrinogen-to-fibrin conversion were completely suppressed in these studies by blockage of the extrinsic system. Our own studies on the gene therapy of sepsis (see below) have shown that blocking tissue factor with antisense strategies can reduce mortality in septic mice. Thus, it is reasonable to conclude that the tissue factor-dependent extrinsic system plays the dominant role in the activation of coagulation in sepsis.

The coagulation system contains several inhibitory systems that are of major importance. Foremost among them are antithrombin III and the protein C–protein S system. The levels of the inhibitor systems are generally depressed in septic patients [30, 68, 173], with antithrombin III levels falling rapidly when sepsis occurs. Mammen et al. [123] observed a 90% mortality in patients whose

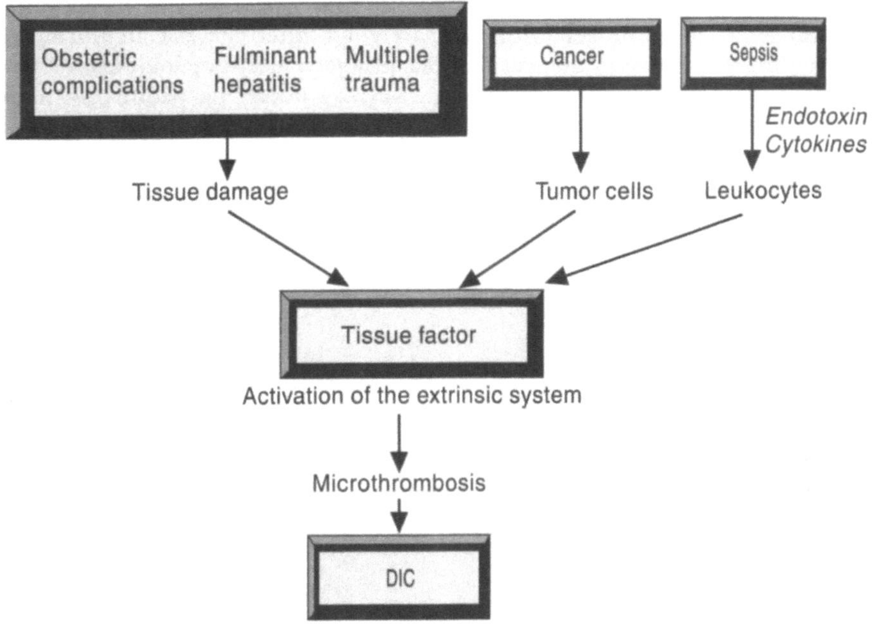

Fig. 7. DIC can be triggered in critically ill and noncritically ill patients (e.g., with malignant tumors) by the release of tissue factor into the circulation

antithrombin III plasma levels fell below 70%. Antithrombin III levels lower than 60% are reportedly associated with 100% mortality. TNF and interleukin 1 induce a down-regulation of thrombomodulin expression on endothelial cells, leading to a decrease in protein C activity [46, 139]. This in turn contributes further to the development of a procoagulant state. Taylor et al. [191] confirmed the importance of the protein C–protein S system in primates exposed to *Escherichia coli*. When the activation of protein C was influenced by the administration of monoclonal antibodies, DIC developed at a ten times lower dose of *Escherichia coli* than in control animals. The authors also found that the administration of activated protein C protected against DIC and organ failure.

Fibrinolytic System

Activation of the fibrinolytic system occurs in septic patients with DIC, with laboratory tests showing reduced plasma levels of fibrinolytic proteins and increased levels of fibrin degradation products. Fibrinolytic activation has generally been interpreted as a secondary process resulting from activated coagulation. Clinical studies in patients suggest that the fibrinolytic system is initially activated and is later inhibited [207]. The injection of endotoxin or TNF in experimental subjects [188, 200] is followed by a rise in tissue- and urokinase-type plasminogen activators, thereby inducing the formation of plasmin from plasminogen. Approximately 1 h after the rise in fibrinolytic activity, there is a rise in the levels of plasminogen activator inhibitor (PAI-1), with complete inhibition of fibrinolytic activity occurring within 3–4 h. Assuming that procoagulant activation is maximal at 4–5 h, it follows that an imbalance of the procoagulant and fibrinolytic systems exists in sepsis. This would account for the incomplete dissolution of fibrin deposits in the microcirculation of septic patients.

Platelets

The platelet count is generally reduced in septic states (see Table 1). This thrombocytopenia results from platelet consumption by fibrin deposits, platelet adhesion to altered endothelial cells, and pulmonary and hepatic sequestration. Generally a close correlation exists between depressed platelet counts and patient mortality. Abnormalities of platelet function are not caused entirely by sepsis per se; they can also occur in the setting of antibiotic therapy, or they may be associated with sepsis-related uremia [73].

Translocation

In recent years increased attention has been given to the importance of translocation through the bowel wall. Shock can disrupt the integrity of the gastrointestinal barrier, allowing the bowel wall to become permeable to bacteria, endotoxin, and other macromolecular complexes. This endotoxin seepage and bacterial translocation from the alimentary tract have been documented in experimental animals, and the gastrointestinal tract has been characterized as the "motor" of multiple organ failure [132]. Some sepsis researchers have even described the gastrointestinal tract as the *undrained abscess* of MOF [126].

Role of the Liver

Among its essential functions, the liver serves to regulate bowel-dependent endotoxemia, the production of inflammatory mediators, and plasma protein synthesis. Interposed between the intestinal and systemic circulations, the liver plays a key role in the reduction or elimination of translocated bacteria and toxins from the intestinal tract. If the liver is unable to perform its clearance function adequately, translocated toxins will enter the systemic circulation. Especially in cases where hepatic dysfunction allows mediators to flood the systemic circulation, the burden passes to the next largest organ of the reticuloendothelial system, the lung. This chain of events highlights the importance of gastrointestinal–liver interactions as well as the "liver–lung axis."

Tissue Oxygenation

The general inflammatory response is accompanied by a cellular hypoxia whose precise cause has been a mystery. Two pathogenic mechanisms have been proposed: the cellular hypoxia may result from microcirculatory failure with inadequate oxygen delivery to the tissues, or it may result from a primary failure of cellular metabolism. Hotchkiss et al. [97] used NMR spectroscopy and isotope techniques in rats to show that the failure of cellular metabolism is a secondary phenomenon, at least in live animal models, indicating that microcirculatory dysfunction is a primary process that initiates the other changes.

Expressed in clinical terms, this means that a marked reduction of tissue oxygenation can be demonstrated in patients with severe sepsis. Despite adequate oxygen delivery in the arterial blood, there is a reduction of oxygen uptake and thus of oxygen consumption in the tissues. Shoemaker [174] considers this latent oxygen debt to be a serious risk factor and advocates increasing oxygen delivery in these patients only as long as a gain in oxygen consumption can be achieved. More recent studies have been unable to confirm a pathologic dependence of oxygen consumption on oxygen delivery [134]. Oxygen delivery and consumption can be measured with a Swan-Ganz catheter, which yields information on pulmonary and systemic vascular resistance in addition to such parameters as pulmonary arterial pressure, pulmonary capillary wedge pressure, and cardiac output.

The hemodynamic response of the organism involves a hyperdynamic reaction at the macrocirculatory level, which some authors have interpreted as an attempt to reestablish adequate tissue oxygenation. One feature of this hyperdynamic phase of sepsis is a paralysis of the peripheral vascular system, characterized by a failure of adequate regulation of blood distribution. A 1992 study by Hollenberg et al. [96] showed that a circulating substance isolated from the serum of septic patients exerted a relaxing effect on the contracted smooth muscle of the aortic ring in rats. Nitric oxide (NO), released locally as "endothelium-derived relaxing factor," functions as the mediator of this arteriolar dilatation [9, 121]. There is a concomitant rise in plasma endothelin levels, representing an ineffectual attempt at vasoconstriction and counter-regulation [135, 206].

Myocardial Dysfunction

Direct myocardial depression is another feature of multiple organ failure in sepsis [211]. A circulating "myocardial depressant factor," first demonstrated by Parrillo et al. in 1985, may be a contributing factor [143]. Parillo treated rat cardiac muscle preparations with serum from a total of 20 patients with septic shock and found that the sera from septic patients depressed myocardial contractility in relation to controls. A more recent study showed that TNF has strong cardiodepressant properties, suggesting that at least one aspect of myocardial depression in septic shock is attributable to this mediator [90].

Treatment of Sepsis (see Table 3)

Surgical Eradication of the Septic Focus

Identification of the primary focus is an important factor in the optimum treatment of sepsis. If a circumscribed focus is present, it should be eliminated or minimized by surgical or interventional means. In septic peritonitis, for example, surgical intervention to eradicate toxin-producing foci will favorably affect the disease process.

Antibiotic Therapy

Diagnostic samples such as blood, urine, CSF, and bronchial secretions should be collected and evaluated before antibiotic treatment is initiated. Specific antibiotic therapy based on identification of the pathogen and sensitivity testing is preferred over nonspecific therapy, but this is rarely feasible for patients who present in the initial phase of sepsis. Thus, initial nonspecific empirical antibiotic treatment should be guided by the potential primary focus, the underlying disease, nosocomial epidemiology, and host resistance status, especially since a potential pathogenic microorganism can be identified in only about one-fourth to one-half of cases.

Table 3. Management of sepsis in ICU patients

Standard therapies	Adjuvant therapies (some experimental)	Experimental approaches
Surgical eradication of septic focus	Antithrombin III administration	Pharmacologic suppression of NO
Antibiotic therapy hemofiltration	Continuous mechanical	Plasmapharesis
Improving oxygenation anti-inflammatory agents	Immunoglobulin administration	Administration of nonsteroidal
Volume replacement	Low-dose hydrocortisone	High-dose naloxone therapy replacement
Catecholamine administration	Administration of C1 esterase inhibitor *	Manipulation at the cytokine level (see text)
Administration of centoxin **	PAF antagonists	

The left column shows the standard treatments. The center column lists the adjuvant therapies practiced by the authors, with (*) indicating use in selected cases and (**) indicating treatments that were discontinued in 1993.
PAF, platelet-activating factor.

Adequate Oxygenation

To improve peripheral oxygen delivery in septic shock, impairment of pulmonary gas exchange is treated by intubating the patient and providing adequate ventilatory therapy. The indication for early ventilatory support is widely acknowledged. Oxygen delivery can also be enhanced by providing appropriate volume replacement and catecholamine therapy to increase the cardiac output. Two recent studies [175, 198] postulate that patient mortality declines as oxygen delivery is increased, while other authors call for moderation when attempting to maximize oxygen delivery [8]. Hayes et al. [89] cautioned in 1994 against maximizing oxygen delivery "at any cost" due to the potential for increased iatrogenic mortality.

Volume Loading

The primary treatment for hypotension in sepsis is volume repletion, using a Swan-Ganz catheter to monitor and direct the therapy [127]. However, generous volume repletion appears to be problematic when capillary leakage is present due to the short intravascular retention time. There is still too little experience with the use of small hypertonic fluid volumes ("small volume resuscitation") to draw definite conclusions [111], although Kreimeier and Messmer achieved positive circulatory effects with hypertonic–hyperoncotic saline dextran solutions administered during continuous endotoxin infusion in laboratory animals [112].

Blood transfusion can not only increase oxygen delivery but can also provide effective volume therapy, for the transfused erythrocytes, unlike other substances, are retained within the intravascular space even when capillary leakage is present. At the latest consensus conference on sepsis held in 1994, it was agreed that the hemoglobin level in septic shock should not be allowed to fall into the range of 7–8 g/dl and should be raised to more than 10 g/dl [176]. Marik and his group emphasized the importance of transfusing relatively fresh packed red blood cells no more than 10 days old to ensure adequate deformability of the transfused cells [124].

Catecholamine Therapy

Catecholaminergic agents can also be administered to promote hemodynamic stabilization in septic shock. Dopamine is usually administered in low doses to provide support of renal function. Dobutamine improves impaired ventricular contractility and increases peripheral oxygen delivery [204]. Norepinephrine, with its predominantly α-adrenergic activity, is the current agent of choice for restoring tone to the peripheral vascular system. Studies from 1987 and 1988 dispelled earlier fears that the vasoconstriction induced by norepinephrine could cause further deterioration of renal function [50, 131]. On the contrary, the norepinephrine-induced rise in blood pressure tends to improve diuresis in patients who have received adequate volume repletion [150].

Antithrombin III Replacement

Antithrombin III functions as an important regulator and inhibitor in the coagulation system. It chiefly inhibits factor Xa and thrombin. The low levels of antithrombin III in septic patients are apparently a result of increased consumption due to hypercoagulability. This provides a rationale for the therapeutic use of antithrombin III products (e.g., Kybernin HS). The results of several animal studies and clinical studies based on small case numbers have already been published. In rats exposed to endotoxin, preliminary treatment with high doses of antithrombin III led to a decrease in intravascular coagulation and organ damage and improved survival [52, 149]. Similar results were reported in primates with sepsis triggered by *E. coli* [59]. In 1985, Blauhut et al. [16] published the first randomized clinical study on the use of antithrombin III (Kybernin HS) in 51 patients with shock and DIC. The treatment group showed a more rapid normalization of coagulation status, although mortality was not improved. In the clinical study of Seitz et al. [170], 29 patients with septic shock received antithrombin III (Kybernin HS) and fresh plasma; 13 of these patients died, compared with 12 of 13 untreated patients. Fourrier et al. [66] reported in 1993 on a placebo-controlled, double-blind study in 35 patients with septic shock. The 44% reduction of mortality in the group treated with antithrombin III replacement was not statistically significant due to the small number of cases, but a marked improvement in sepsis-induced DIC was apparent in the group that received antithrombin III. Jochum and his group [7, 103, 138] recommend raising the antithrombin III level into the range of 140% for up to 4 days in patients with septic shock or multiple injuries. This requires a total infusion of approximately 18 000 U of antithrombin III per patient. Vinazzer [202] reported recently on his experience with antithrombin III replacement in shock. He states that the antithrombin III level in shock should not be allowed to fall below 80%, and that this measure will significantly reduce the duration of DIC. Vinazzer notes, however, that antithrombin III doses should be administered frequently in acute DIC, since the usual half-life of 2.5 days may be shortened to less than 4 h. In our department we follow Vinazzer's recommendations in the treatment of patients with septic shock and try to maintain an antithrombin III level of 80%.

Fibrinolytic Agents

Lorente and his group [120] were able to show that the imbalance between the activation of coagulation and the inhibition of fibrinolysis plays an essential role in sepsis. Lorente found that patients who did not survive showed a markedly greater activation of coagulation than patients who survived. Accordingly, there was a significantly greater inhibition of fibrinolysis in the patients who did not survive. Such findings support the use of fibrinolytic therapy in patients with septic shock in order to correct the imbalance and its consequences [41]. Streptokinase administered to rats with endotoxemia increased the survival rate from 8% to 70% [179], demonstrating the importance of fibrinolysis for the survival of the animals. The administration of fibrinolytic agents in pigs with induced trauma prevented the development of acute lung injury [85]. Initial clinical experience is already available on the use of fibrinolytic agents in patients with acute respiratory distress syndrome (ARDS), which also is associated with microthrombosis in the pulmonary vascular tree [84, 86, 87].

Nutrition and Digestive Decontamination

Given the central role of the bowel in the perpetuation of sepsis, one can appreciate the primary importance of nutrition in the critically ill patient. Increased attention has been paid to the importance of nutrition for the immune system in recent years. Recent authors have advocated the earliest possible initiation of enteral feeding, as opposed to long-term parenteral nutrition, to preserve the integrity of the digestive tract [136], with persistent gastroparesis necessitating the use of duodenal and jejunal tubes. Besides the usual nutrients and trace elements, the addition of special supplements has assumed greater importance. Supplementation with omega-3 fatty acids and arginine improves the postoperative course in patients placed on early enteral feeding [48]. A multicenter study in 326 ICU patients, published in 1995, showed that enteral supplementation with arginine, nucleotides, and fish oil was associated with a significantly lower incidence of acquired infections as well as a significantly reduced hospital stay [29]. It has also been shown that adding glutamine to the parenteral diet can help shorten hospitalization by reducing intestinal atrophy and lowering the overall incidence of infection [197, 215]. These approaches have given rise to the term *immunonutrition*.

Following the initial 1984 study by Stoutenbeek et al. [187], attempts have been made, especially in Europe, to sterilize the gastrointestinal tract by the administration of nonabsorbable antibiotics as a means of preventing endogenous microorganisms from becoming pathogenic. This therapy, known as selective decontamination of the digestive tract (SDD), has been the subject of numerous recent controlled studies. While most of these studies have shown a reduction in pneumonia rates, generally they have not shown improvement in mortality [40, 47, 62, 71, 83, 148]. Prophylactic SDD cannot prevent bacterial translocation in the gastrointestinal tract and may actually promote the translocation of gram-positive organisms [100].

Inhibition of Nitric Oxide

For several years there has been a new pharmacologic approach to the treatment of hypotension in septic shock. It is assumed that mediator-dependent vasodilatation and hypotension are induced by the release of local nitric oxide (NO). In animal models of sepsis, increased concentrations of NO in exhaled gas have been detected as an early marker of pulmonary inflammation [186]. Thus, the inhibition of this increased NO synthesis by various arginine derivatives holds promise as a therapeutic approach. Initial positive findings have been reported in animal studies [28], and NO synthetase inhibitors have been successfully used in small numbers of patients [118, 114, 165]. On the other hand, patients who have developed respiratory failure with ARDS during the course of sepsis may benefit from the inhalation of NO, whose short physiologic half-life of several seconds effectively limits the effects of the gas to the lung [154].

Corticosteroids

The early administration of high doses of corticoids such as methylprednisolone in septic shock is not supported by the results of two multicenter studies conducted in 1987 [26, 193]. The mortality rates in these studies were not lowered by corticoid therapy and in fact were increased due to secondary complications. In 1991, Rothwell [158] published a clinical study using ACTH stimulation to show that a relative adrenocortical insufficiency exists in patients with septic shock, suggesting that replacement with physiologic doses of hydrocortisone should be of therapeutic benefit. Several groups have already reported positive clinical results, consisting mainly of hemodynamic improvement, by employing this approach [31, 33, 166]. Since these studies, Briegel et al. [32] have shown experimentally that hydrocortisone reduces the substantial increase in phospholipase A_2 activity that occurs in sepsis.

Free-Radical Scavengers

The sequence of events in septic shock leads to neutrophil activation with the generation of oxygen-derived free radicals that overwhelm normal antioxidant defenses, resulting in lipid peroxidation and tissue injury [76]. N-acetylcysteine is a known antioxidant and free-radical scavenger that acts mainly via the glutathione system. In recent studies, the use of N-acetylcysteine in sepsis has yielded positive results in dogs [5] and in human patients [151, 181]. An initial prospective study in 66 patients suggests that this agent may also be beneficial in ARDS [101]. Animal studies have shown that N-acetylcysteine can largely prevent pulmonary fibrin deposition in DIC [209].

Lazaroids belonging to the class of 21-aminosteroids are among the newest free-radical scavengers. One agent, tirilazad, has been available for use in several European countries since March of 1995. So far there have been no reports on the use of tirilazad in septic patients, but positive experimental results in mice [172], rats [119], dogs [104], and calves [171] suggest that tirilazad would be beneficial in septic patients.

Naloxone

In 1978, Holaday and Faden [94] interpreted hypotension in septic shock as a "flooding" of the organism with endogenous opiates. This prompted attempts to use the opiate antagonist naloxone as a means of antagonizing sepsis-related hypotension. Naloxone produced a dose-dependent blood pressure reduction in rats with endotoxic shock, showing maximum efficacy at doses in excess of 1 mg/kg [94]. Holaday ascribed similar pressor effects to thyrotropin-releasing hormone (TRH) in rats with endotoxic shock [95]. To date, however, neither naloxone [82] nor TRH has achieved clinical importance.

Hemofiltration

Continuous hemofiltration can be used for fluid management in septic patients, and continuous hemodiafiltration is particularly useful for eliminating uremic substances in hemodynamically unstable patients. Continuous mechanical hemofiltration has been used increasingly in recent years as an extracorporeal technique for removing mediators of small and intermediate molecular size. Gomez showed in 1990 that hemofiltration could reverse left ventricular dysfunction in dogs with induced sepsis [75], leading him to postulate the elimination of a "myocardial depressant factor" by hemofiltration. Stein achieved similar positive results the same year with continuous hemofiltration in pigs [183]. A later study showed that the degree of improvement in ventricular contractility correlates directly with an increase in filtrate volume [78]. Since then, several groups of authors have shown that continuous hemofiltration effectively eliminates both TNF and interleukin 1 [12, 195] with no removal of endotoxin and very little removal of interleukin 6. The ability of the hemofiltration membrane to remove platelet-activating factor has also been shown [157]. So far, however, it has been difficult to determine the proportion of the eliminated substances in relation to the total endogenous pool. Our own experience shows that positive effects are achieved even in the early phase of sepsis, and we feel that continuous mechanical venovenous hemofiltration should be started early in patients who still have intact renal function. Temperature reduction by the extracorporeal system has proved to be an important side benefit of this therapy, and generally the body temperature falls into the normal range. We still know little about the capabilities of plasmapheresis as an effective extracorporeal technique for toxin elimination [147].

Treatments That Act on Mediators

Another therapeutic approach involves the use of nonsteroidal anti-inflammatory agents that act on the arachidonic acid metabolism and modify the activity of cyclooxygenase and lipooxygenase. Both indomethacin and ibuprofen have been found to reduce mortality in septic laboratory animals, although their value in the treatment of septic patients is less clear [22, 65].

The intravenous administration of specific antibodies could also have positive effects. In a large trial in more than 543 patients, Ziegler [214] showed that the administration of a human monoclonal IgM antibody against the lipid-A structure of endotoxin could reduce mortality from sepsis. This effect was limited to the subset of patients with gram-negative bacteremia, however. Greenman, in a second multicenter study, achieved similar results with a mouse antibody [77]. The product Centoxin, previously approved for use in Germany, was withdrawn in January 1993, after an American phase III study in patients without gram-negative bacteremia showed a higher death rate than in a placebo-treated group. Bactericidal/permeability-increasing protein (BPI) may provide an alternative approach based on its ability to bind and neutralize endotoxin [125]. Initial animal studies with BPI have yielded promising results [64, 102].

The therapeutic options that are available for treating sepsis at the cytokine level are summarized below. TNF is considered a central mediator of sepsis. The neutralization of endogenously released TNF by monoclonal antibodies has lowered mortality in experimental animals [92, 163]. Protective effects of TNF must be considered in interpreting these results, however [161]. Based on the promising results of an initial pilot study in patients [205], multicenter studies were launched in Europe and the U.S. to test the efficacy of antibodies against TNF in sepsis [1]. The results of these studies were disappointing, however; only the subset of septic patients with high levels of interleukin 6 appeared to benefit. This has prompted a supplemental multicenter study, now in progress, on TNF antibodies that are administered strictly to patients with high interleukin 6 levels. The phosphodiesterase inhibitor pentoxifylline, used in the treatment of arterial insufficiency, significantly reduced TNF production in controlled endotoxemia in humans [213], inducing a partial blockage of the endogenous TNF response. This may provide a rationale for the use of pentoxifylline in sepsis [194], although recent animal studies suggest that this drug must be administered during a relatively early "therapeutic window" to avoid adverse effects in patients with fully established septic shock [153].

The use of interleukin-1 receptor antagonists also yielded promising results in initial animal studies [2], but clinical multicenter studies [63] were as dis-

---

Methods of treating sepsis at the cytokine level	• **Antibodies against cytokines:**
	  – TNF antibody
	  – Interleukin-6 antibody
	
	• **Antibodies against cytokine receptors:**
	  – Interleukin-1 receptor antibody
	
	• **Cytokine receptor antagonist:**
	  – Interleukin-1 receptor antagonist
	
	• **Circulating inhibitors:**
	  – Interleukin-1 inhibitor
	  – Interleukin-6 inhibitor
	  – TNF inhibitor

---

appointing as the anti-TNF studies. Likewise, clinical multicenter studies using antagonists against platelet-activating factor showed no improvement in mortality [51], and this concept of antagonizing a single mediator does not appear to be rewarding.

The above approaches are aimed strictly at the cytokine class of mediators, but sepsis also involves the activation of various other cascades such as the complement system [53], which is regulated by its own enzyme inhibitor. Guerrero et al. [79] found that the exogenous administration of this C1-esterase inhibitor prevented endotoxin-induced pulmonary dysfunction in dogs. This suggests that replacement of this inhibitor may offer an approach to the treatment of sepsis in human patients [80, 81, 140].

Polyvalent Immunoglobulins

Since the therapeutic modification or blockage of a single mediator has not proved effective, the administration of polyvalent immunoglobulins may offer a more promising approach. These substances provide the organism with a number of antibodies and improve opsonization. In 1991, Dominioni [55] and Schedel [164] published two prospective, randomized double-blind studies on the high-dose parenteral administration of polyclonal and polyvalent immunoglobulins for the purpose of neutralizing endotoxin. This type of therapy led to a significant reduction of mortality in adult patients with sepsis. A more recent study by Pilz et al. [146] on polyvalent immunoglobulin therapy after cardiac surgery showed a marked reduction of mortality and an improvement in prognosis.

Our Therapeutic Approach

In 1991, we adopted a combined treatment regimen for sepsis at our ICU consisting of the administration of polyvalent IgM-enriched immunoglobulins and low-dose hydrocortisone. The basic principles of these therapies were detailed above. By August of 1994, we had used this regimen in a total of 64 patients who had undergone general or cardiac surgery and fulfilled the criteria for septic shock [18]. Treatment included epinephrine or norepinephrine administered at $\geq$ 0.2 µg/kg body weight/min following adequate volume replacement. An initial bolus injection of 100 mg hydrocortisone was given over a period of 15 min, followed by continuous infusion at a rate of 200–300 mg/day [33]. The IgM-enriched immunoglobulin preparation was administered in a dose of 15 g/day for 3 days. Patients were classified as *responders* if their catecholamine dose could be reduced by one-half within 24 h. Most of the patients in our study stabilized while on this regimen. A total of 47 patients (73%) met the criteria for responders, while 17 patients were classified as *nonresponders*. The mortality rate in the nonresponder group was 76% versus only 23% in the responder group ($p<0.001$). There was no difference in initial APACHE-II scores between the two groups. We conclude from these results that the combined regimen is a very promising approach in the adjuvant treatment of sepsis.

Any effective sepsis therapy in ICU patients must be based on a standard program that is instituted as soon as the diagnosis is made. We feel that adjuvant measures should be started early, and that such a regimen is not indicated for moribund patients who are admitted with advanced shock. General ICU management should include appropriate monitoring protocols (e.g., continuous measurement of cardiac output), early enteral feeding (e.g., immunonutrition with supplemental arginine and omega-3 fatty acids), and sedation (e.g., with ketamine [70, 190]). All standard and adjuvant therapies should be administered by competent personnel; this is essential when dealing with a disease like septic shock, which has a general mortality rate of 40%–60%.

Gene Therapy of Sepsis

In the belief that tissue-factor expression plays an essential role in sepsis, we experimented with intravenous somatic gene transfer in mice prior to the induction of sepsis. The study was performed on 180 female BALB/c mice 12 weeks old [19]. The animals were divided into five dose groups in which 1, 1.5, 1.75, 1.875, or 2 µg of endotoxin per mouse was administered by intraperitoneal injection; each animal simultaneously received 15 mg of galactosamine. Twenty-four hours before administration of the endotoxin, the 36 animals in each dose group underwent intravenous somatic gene transfer with 30 µg DNA dissolved in 100 µg lipofectin. For the gene transfer, mouse tissue factor was cloned in an expression vector in the sense orientation (overexpression of biologically active tissue factor), in the antisense orientation (blockage of tissue-factor expression), or as truncated sense cDNA in the wrong reading frame (no change in tissue-factor expression). It was found that tissue-factor expression in the animals treated with antisense TF was significantly less than in the other two groups. Additionally, the antisense group showed almost no evidence of fibrin deposition in the kidney and other organs, whereas the other animals, especially the sense group, showed prominent fibrin deposits. As for survival, the suppression of tissue-factor induction by intravenous somatic gene transfer shifted the endotoxin-induced mortality curve to the right, and animals treated with antisense TF showed a significantly higher survival rate than the animals in the other groups. Our findings indicate that the antisense method offers a promising new approach in the treatment of sepsis.

Since tissue-factor expression is regulated by the transcription factors nuclear factor κB (NFκB) and activator protein 1 (AP1) [112], we sought to determine whether sepsis-related mortality in mice could be reduced by influencing these transcription factors [20], i.e., by using the inhibitor IκB to block NFκB and using mutated jun to block AP1. A total of 48 female BALB/c mice aged 12 weeks were used in the study. The animals were divided into four groups and underwent an intravenous somatic gene transfer with 30 µg DNA dissolved in 100 µg lipofectin. Animals in group 1 received only the expression vector. For the gene transfer in group 2, IκB was cloned in an expression vector in the sense orientation for overexpression of biologically active inhibitor. Mutated jun was overexpressed in the group 3 animals, and both IκB and mutated jun were overexpressed in group 4. Twenty-four hours after the gene transfer, 1.75 µg endotoxin was administered intraperitoneally in all animals along with 15 mg of galactosamine. We found that inhibition of the transcription factors NFκB and AP1 led to a significant reduction of 24-h mortality in the experimental animals. The fact that the overexpression of IκB and mutated jun reduced sepsis-related mortality in the mouse model proves that the transcription factors NFκB and AP1 play an important role in sepsis.

Fulminant Forms of Sepsis

Meningococcal Sepsis

Fulminant meningococcal sepsis, which generally occurs in children and is less common in adults, is a hyperacute meningococcal infection that is almost always fatal. Cases with concomitant bilateral adrenal hemorrhage are classified as Waterhouse-Friderichsen syndrome, after the researchers who described the pathologic features of the syndrome between 1911 and 1918.

Fulminant meningococcal sepsis is associated with generalized petechial hemorrhages, purpura, and shock necessitating volume replacement and vasopressor therapy. Capillary leakage and myocardial dysfunction are also present. Bilateral adrenal hemorrhage initially points to acute adrenal insufficiency as the cause of the shock, but this appears to be true only in a certain percentage of cases. Some authors relate fulminant meningococcal sepsis to the Sanarelli-Shwartzman reaction, in which two separate endotoxin injections in experimental animals are followed by coagulopathy and necrotic skin lesions.

Meningococcal sepsis has a particularly high association with thrombocytopenia and the development of DIC, with petechiae and ecchymoses noted at bedside examination. While low antithrombin III levels are a prominent finding in adults with meningococcal sepsis, children show a more pronounced decline in protein C and protein S. Leclerc et al. [114] not only found marked reductions of protein C and S in children with shock and DIC, but they also showed that the initial levels were a useful prognostic indicator of patient survival: mortality was significantly higher in children with low initial levels of protein C and S. McManus [129] also found a significant correlation between mortality and coagulation abnormalities in children with meningococcal sepsis. Besides the use of antibiotics and catecholamines, volume repletion with fresh plasma has generally been advocated in the acute stage of meningococcal sepsis to ensure a balanced supply of coagulation factors. More recent studies from Scandinavia indicate, however, that the administration of fresh plasma may adversely affect patient outcomes [37].

Sepsis After Splenectomy: the OPSI Syndrome

In recent decades cases of severe, usually fatal sepsis have been reported after splenectomy, first in children and later in adults. The term "overwhelming postsplenectomy infection syndrome" (OPSI syndrome) has been applied to this condition [17, 61, 69, 162]. Patients with OPSI syndrome have fulminant clinical symptoms marked by fever, nausea, obtundation, and signs of DIC, with death often occurring within a few hours. The pathogenesis is based on a postsplenectomy disturbance of phagocytosis in the reticuloendotheilal system. The tetrapeptide tuftsin, produced in the spleen, appears to play an important role in this process. The risk of developing OPSI syndrome persists for life in patients who have undergone splenectomy. Since the pathogenesis rests mainly on pneumococcal infection, inoculation with pneumococcal vaccine is recommended in splenectomized patients [130].

Acute Respiratory Distress Syndrome

Moderate and severe forms of SIRS may progress to established respiratory failure [98] through a process of secondary or indirect lung injury. Cytokines play a major role in the pathogenesis of this secondary lung injury, and their pulmonary effects have been well documented in animal models [60, 184]. Only a slight elevation of circulating cytokines may be found in patients with overt ARDS, but bronchoalveolar lavage (BAL) will demonstrate high cytokine levels in this condition [177, 189]. This is consistent with earlier comments on the "lung–liver axis" and the clearance function of the lung in removing toxins and mediators.

Definition of ARDS

The latest American-European Consensus Conference on ARDS, held in 1992, recommended three main criteria for the definition of ARDS (preferring the term "acute" rather than "adult" as a descriptor for the syndrome):

Diagnostic evaluation of DIC in the intensive care unit	
	• **Clinical features of DIC**
	• Platelet count ↓
	• Partial thromboplastin time (PTT) ↑
	• Prothrombin time ↑ (Quick PT ↓)
	• Fibrinogen ↓
	• Thrombin time ↑ (especially in DIC with reactive hyperfibrinolysis)
	• Antithrombin III ↓
	• Fibrin monomers ↑
	• Thrombin-antithrombin III complex (TAT) ↑
	• Fibrinopeptide A ↑
	• Prothrombin fragments (F_{1+2}) ↑
	• Fibrin(ogen) degradation products ↑ (in DIC with reactive hyperfibrinolysis)
	• D-dimer ↑ (in DIC with reactive hyperfibrinolysis)

1. With regard to oxygenation, the ratio of arterial oxygen tension to inspired oxygen fraction, PaO_2/FIO_2, must be ≤ 200 mm Hg in ARDS. A ratio ≤ 300 mg Hg is sufficient for acute lung injury (ALI).
2. Bilateral pulmonary infiltrates must be visible on the frontal chest radiograph.
3. The pulmonary wedge pressure must be ≤ 18 mm Hg to exclude primary cardiologic disease.

Numerous predisposing factors may be involved in the development of ARDS. These include direct insults (e.g., trauma, aspiration, inhalation injury) as well as indirect effects (e.g., due to sepsis or pancreatitis).

Besides the chest radiograph, computed tomography (CT) has assumed increasing importance in the diagnosis of ARDS. CT often shows focal densities primarily in the dependent regions of the lungs, with advanced cases of ARDS still showing a 10%–20% proportion of healthy lung tissue, which Gattinoni calls "baby lung" [72]. These residual healthy lung areas are exceptionally sensitive to ventilation-induced pressure and volume trauma.

Pathologic Changes in ARDS

Once the clinical picture has progressed to fully established ARDS, the pathologic changes in the lung are indistinguishable from those of primary respiratory failure. Light microscopic examination in the early phase shows swelling of the pulmonary capillaries with an accumulation of proteinaceous fluid in the alveolar spaces and interstitium. Within this fluid, hyaline membranes form in the alveoli. Erythrocytes and neutrophils are found in the air-filled spaces, and thrombi and fibrin deposits cause variable occlusion of pulmonary capillaries. This early phase lasts 1-3 days. In rabbits with experimental lung injury, Sitrin et al. [178] demonstrated extensive intra-alveolar fibrin production and found that intravenously administered radiolabeled fibrinogen accumulated in the lung parenchyma. Concomitant BAL demonstrated a high procoagulant activity in the lavage fluid. In patients with ARDS, Idell et al. [99] also found high procoagulant activity in BAL samples due mainly to the presence of tissue factor and factor VII. Fibrinolytic activity could not be demonstrated in the BAL of these patients. As early as 1976, Bone et al. [25] demonstrated a close relationship between ARDS and DIC, with a total of 23% of ARDS patients developing DIC. A detailed review of the role of the coagulation system in ARDS was last published in a 1994 issue of *Chest* [88]. The early phase of ARDS is followed by the proliferative phase, characterized by persistent fluid accumulation in the alveoli and interstitium accompanied by epithelial proliferation within the alveoli. The final phase is a fibrotic transformation in which the hyaline membranes regress and fibroblasts proliferate in the alveolar spaces.

Treatment of ARDS

Since causal treatment for ARDS is not yet available, the goal of therapeutic measures is to support cellular and physiologic functions (e.g., gas exchange, organ perfusion, and aerobic metabolism) until the lung injury has resolved [109, 155, 156]. The foremost measure is mechanical ventilatory support with tidal volumes limited to 6–10 ml/kg body weight and an upper pressure limit no higher than 35 cm H_2O. It is desirable to reduce the inspired oxygen concentration to ≤ 0.6, and the positive end-expiratory pressure should be adjusted to provide optimum oxygen delivery. Permissive hypercapnia may be allowed to avoid further pressure and volume injury to the lung.

Because the regional pulmonary changes in ARDS mainly involve the dependent, posterior lung regions, prone positioning can be a useful therapeutic adjunct [93]. Indeed, prone positioning has become a standard part of the therapy of ARDS, and a large percentage of patient respond to this measure with an acute improvement in oxygenation. Moving the ventilated patient to the prone position converts the posterior lung areas into nondependent areas, leading to an acute improvement in the ventilation–perfusion ratio. This position also promotes the mobilization of airway secretions.

Another standard component of ARDS therapy is fluid restriction. Consistent with hydrostatic principles, induced intravascular hypovolemia provides a very effective method of eliminating accumulated extravascular lung water. Thus, diuretics are among the standard medications used in the therapy of ARDS. If taken to an extreme, fluid restriction can lead to perfusion deficits and induction of iatrogenic shock [168].

The possibility of NO inhalation therapy in ARDS was previously noted. Inspiratory NO concentrations of 5–80 ppm are generally used in this type of therapy. Several commercial systems for NO inhalation therapy have become available, although there have been no controlled clinical studies on their use in ARDS. The inhalation of aerosolized prostacyclin has also been used in the treatment of ARDS; Walmrath et al. [208] have reported on the successful use of this therapy in three patients. In contrast to infants with IRDS (infant respiratory distress syndrome), adult patients with ARDS do not have a primary surfactant deficiency, so surfactant replacement in ARDS patients has become a controversial issue [116].

Several extracorporeal techniques are available for supporting gas exchange in ARDS. The intravenous oxygenator (IVOX), which is introduced surgically into the superior and inferior vena cava, has been successfully used at several institutions [91], although clinical trials are still pending. Extracorporeal membrane oxygenation (ECMO) is widely used in neonatology and pediatrics for various causes of respiratory failure and involves cannulation of the internal jugular vein and carotid artery. Venovenous extracorporeal CO_2 removal ($ECCO_2R$) has yielded good results in adult ARDS patients, especially at European centers.

Newer therapeutic strategies still in the experimental stage involve the use of gene transfer to prevent secondary lung injury. Conary et al. [45], for example, induced hyperexpression of the prostaglandin synthase enzyme in rabbits by the intravenous transfusion of cDNA. This led to an increased production of prostacyclin and prostaglandin E2 and a marked reduction of endotoxin-induced thromboxane release and pulmonary hypertension in the treated animals. This confirms the feasibility of protecting the lungs from secondary endotoxin injury by the hyperexpression of certain genes.

Obstetric Complications

Acute coagulation disorders in obstetrics can have various causes. In particular, placental abruption and amniotic fluid embolism have been implicated in the development of DIC. Large retroplacental hematomas generally lead to fetal death, and early uterine evacuation is the primary means of achieving adequate hemostasis. Intrauterine retention of the dead fetus tends to exacerbate shock and can perpetuate DIC.

Amniotic fluid embolism results from the entry of amniotic fluid into the maternal circulation, leading to cardiorespiratory failure and coagulopathy. Clinically, patients manifest respiratory insufficiency with dyspnea and cyanosis. Neurologic symptoms range from confusion and motor unrest to seizures. Fetal hairs, vernix caseosa, and mucin can be detected in the lung and right heart. Severe coagulopathy with a bleeding diathesis develops within 30 min to several hours after the embolic event. The severity of the coagulation disorder does not correlate with the amount of material that has embolized to the lung [117]. The exact pathogenic mechanism of DIC in amniotic fluid embolism is unknown. It may relate to particle constituents as well as unidentified activators in the amniotic fluid. Besides symptomatic treatment of shock and the coagulopathy, early evacuation of the uterus is an important part of management.

General Treatment Recommendations for DIC

Given the diverse etiologies of DIC, general therapeutic strategies must focus on correction of the underlying problem and especially on general intensive care. Consideration must also be given to the staffing of the ICU, since the presence of competent critical care physicians can improve patient outcomes in septic shock [152]. An important basic factor in the treatment of DIC is repletion of the deficient inhibitor potential. The antithrombin III level should be raised to 80% and should be checked several times daily due to the shor-

General recommendations for the treatment of DIC in the ICU	• General intensive care • Antithrombin III replacement (to 80%) • Administration of fresh plasma • Up to 5000 U of heparin/day, as required • Platelet concentrates as required • Packed RBCs as required

tened half-life of antithrombin III in DIC. The administration of fresh plasma provides a source of additional coagulation inhibitors. As early as 1975, Lasch and Heene advocated the use of heparin in overt DIC [113]. Today heparin therapy in DIC is somewhat controversial, although low doses up to 5000 IU/ day appear to be acceptable. Theoretical considerations provide a clear rationale for heparin use during the development of thrombocytopenia, when platelet factor 4, liberated by platelet destruction, neutralizes endogenous heparin and thus negates the efficacy of antithrombin III replacement. An increasing bleeding tendency with overt thrombocytopenia requires repletion with platelet concentrates and may necessitate the transfusion of packed red blood cells.

References

1. Abraham E, Wunderink R, Silverman H, Perl TM, Nasraway S, Levy H, Bone R, Wenzel RP, Balk R, Allred R, Pennington JE, Wherry JC (1995) Efficacy and safety of monoclonal antibody to human tumor necrosis factor alpha in patients with sepsis syndrome: A randomized, controlled, double-blind, multicenter clinical trial. JAMA 273:934–941
2. Alexander HR, Doherty GM, Venzon DJ, Merino MJ, Fraker DL, Norton JA (1992) Recombinant interleukin-1 receptor antagonist (IL-1ra) effective therapy against gram-negative sepsis in rats. Surgery 112:188–193
3. American College of Chest Physicians/Society of Critical Care Medicine Consensus Conference (1992) Definitons for sepsis and organ failure and guidelines for the use of innovative therapies in sepsis. Crit Care Med 20:864–874
4. Anderson BO, Bensard DD, Harken AH (1991) The role of platelet activating factor and its antagonists in shock, sepsis and multiple organ failure. Surgery 172:415–424
5. Bakker J, Zhang H, Depierreux M, van Asbeck S, Vincent JL (1994) Effects of N-acetylcysteine in endotoxic shock. J Crit Care 9:236–243
6. Balk RA, Parrillo JE (1992) Prognostic factors in sepsis. The cold facts [editorial]. Crit Care Med 20:1373–1374
7. Bardenheuer M, Obertacke U, Kleinschmidt C, Scherer R, Eisold C, Jochum M, SchmidtNeuerburg KP (1994) Prophylactic continuous application of antithrombin-III (140% serum activity for 4 days after trauma) for reduction of shock related complications and pulmonary microvascular permeability – A prospective clinical study [abstract]. Intensive Care Med 20 [Suppl 1]:S121
8. Barone JE, Lowenfels AB (1992) Maximization of oxygen delivery: A plea for moderation. J Trauma 33:651–653
9. Battafarano RJ, Dunn DL (1992) Role of nitric oxide during sepsis [editorial]. Crit Care Med 20:1504–1505
10. Baue AE (1992) The Horror autotoxicus and multiple-organ failure. Arch Surg 127:1451–1462
11. Baumgartner JD, Büla C, Vaney C, Wu MM, Eggimann P, Perret C (1992) A novel score for predicting the mortality of septic shock patients. Crit Care Med 20:953–960
12. Bellomo R, Tipping P, Boyce N (1993) Continuous veno-venous hemofiltration with dialysis removes cytokines from the circulation of septic patients. Crit Care Med 21:522–526
13. Benjamin E, Leibowitz AB, Oropello J, Iberti TJ (1992) Systemic hypoxic and inflammatory syndrome: An alternative designation for "sepsis syndrome". Crit Care Med 20:680–682
14. Bernard GR, Artigas A, Brigham KL, Carlet J, Falke K, Hudson L, Lamy M, LeGall JR, Morris A, Spragg R, and the Consensus Committee (1994) The American-European consensus conference on ARDS: definitions, mechanisms, relevant outcomes, and clinical trial coordination. Am J Respir Crit Care Med 149:818–824

15. Biemond BJ, Levi M, ten Cate H, Soule HR, Morris LD, Foster DL, Bogowitz CA, van der Poll T, Büller HR, ten Cate JW (1995) Complete inhibition of endotoxin-induced coagulation activation in chimpanzees with a monoclonal Fab fragment against factor VII/VIIa. Thromb Haemost 73:223–230
16. Blauhut B, Kramar H, Vinazzer H, Bergmann H (1985) Substitution of antithrombin III in shock and DIC: A randomized study. Thromb Res 39:81–89
17. Böhmer R, Ostendorf PC (1987) Aktueller Wissensstand zur Pathogenese und Prophylaxe der Postsplenektomiesepsis (OPSI). Internist 28:777–782
18. Böhrer H, Schmidt H, Bach A, Böttiger BW, Motsch J, Martin E (1995) Combination treatment of sepsis with polyvalent immunoglobulins and low-dose hydrocortisone [abstract]. Crit Care Med 23:A156
19. Böhrer H, Zhang Y, Nawroth PP, Bach A, Böttiger BW, Schmidt H, Martin E (1995) Intravenous somatic gene transfer with antisense tissue factor reduces mortality in mice with endotoxin-induced sepsis [abstract]. Crit Care Med 23:A155
20. Böhrer H, Zhang Y, Qiu F, Nawroth PP, Bach A, Schmidt H, Martin E (1995) Endotoxininduzierte Transkriptionsfaktoren vermitteln die Sepsis-Letalität im Mausmodell [abstract]. Anaesthesist 44 [Suppl 1]:S87
21. Bolton CF, Young GB, Zochodne DW (1993) The neurological complications of sepsis. Ann Neurol 33:94–100
22. Bone RC (1992) Phospholipids and their inhibitors: A critical evaluation of their role in the treatment of sepsis. Crit Care Med 20:884–890
23. Bone RC (1992) Sepsis and coagulation. An important link [editorial]. Chest 101:594–596
24. Bone RC (1992) Toward an epidemiology and natural history of SIRS (systemic inflammatory response syndrome). JAMA 268:3452–3455
25. Bone RC, Francis PB, Pierce AK (1976) Intravascular coagulation associated with the adult respiratory distress syndrome. Am J Med 61:585–589
26. Bone RC, Fisher CJ, Clemmer TP, Slotman GJ, Metz CA, Balk RA, The Methylprednisolone Severe Sepsis Study Group (1987) A controlled clinical trial of high-dose methylprednisolone in the treatment of severe sepsis and septic shock. N Engl J Med 317:653–658
27. Bone RC, Sprung CL, Sibbald WJ (1992) Definitions for sepsis and organ failure [editorial]. Crit Care Med 20:724–726
28. Booke M, Meyer J, Lingnau W, Hinder F, Traber LD, Traber DL (1995) Use of nitric oxide synthase inhibitors in animal models of sepsis. New Horizons 3:123–138
29. Bower RH, Cerra FB, Bershadsky B, Licari JJ, Hoyt DB, Jensen GL, Van Buren CT, Rothkopf MM, Daly JM, Adelsberg BR (1995) Early enteral administration of a formula (Impact) supplemented with arginine, nucleotides, and fish oil in intensive care unit patients: Results of a multicenter, prospective, randomized, clinical trial. Crit Care Med 23:436–449
30. Brandtzaeg P, Sandset PM, Joo GB, Ovstebo R, Abildgaard U, Kierulf P (1989) The quantitative association of plasma endotoxin, antithrombin, protein C, extrinsic pathway inhibitor and fibrinopeptide A in systemic meningococcal disease. Thromb Res 55:459–470
31. Briegel J, Forst H, Kellermann W, Haller M, Peter K (1992) Haemodynamic improvement in refractory septic shock with cortisol replacement therapy [letter]. Intensive Care Med 18:318
32. Briegel J, Kellermann W, Bittl M, Forst H, Hoffmann G, Haller M, Peter K (1992) Influence of physiological doses of hydrocortisone on phospholipase A2 activity in early septic shock [abstract]. Anesthesiology 77:A256
33. Briegel J, Kellermann W, Forst H, Haller M, Bittl M, Hoffmann GE, Büchler M, Uhl W, Peter K and the Phospholipase A2 Study Group (1994) Low-dose hydrocortisone infusion attenuates the systemic inflammatory response syndrome. Clin Investigator 72:782–787
34. Brox JH, Osterud B, Bjorklid E, Fenton JW (1984) Production and availability of thromboplastin in endothelial cells: the effects of thrombin, endotoxin and platelets. Br J Haematol 57:239–246

35. Bull BS, Bull MH (1994) Hypothesis: Disseminated intravascular inflammation as the inflammatory counterpart to disseminated intravascular coagulation. Proc Natl Acad Sci USA 91:8190–8194

36. Burke-Gaffney A, Keenan AK (1993) Modulation of human endothelial cell permeability by combinations of the cytokines interleukin-1/ß, tumor necrosis factor-α, and interferon-γ. Immunopharmacology 25:1–9

37. Busund R, Straume B, Revhaug A (1993) Fatal course in severe meningococcemia: Clinical predictors and effect of transfusion therapy. Crit Care Med 21:1699–1705

38. Carson SD, Johnson DR, Tracy SM (1993) Tissue factor and the extrinsic pathway of coagulation during infection and vascular inflammation. Eur Heart J 14 [Suppl K]:98–104

39. Casey LC, Balk RA, Bone RC (1993) Plasma cytokine and endotoxin levels correlate with survival in patients with the sepsis syndrome. Ann Intern Med 119:771–778

40. Cerra FB, Maddaus MA, Dunn DL, Wells CL, Konstantinides NN, Lehmann SL, Mann HJ (1992) Selective gut decontamination reduces nosocomial infections and length of stay but not mortality or organ failure in surgical intensive care unit patients. Arch Surg 127:163–169

41. Chandler WL (1991) Treatment of thrombosis associated with septic shock [editorial]. J Lab Clin Med 118:513–514

42. Clauss M, Gerlach M, Gerlach H, Brett J, Wang F, Familetti PC, Pan YCE, Olander JV, Connolly DT, Stern D (1990) Vascular permeability factor: A tumor-derived polypeptide that induces endothelial cell and monocyte procoagulant activity, and promotes monocyte migration. J Exp Med 172:1535–1545

43. Clemmer TP, Fisher CJ, Bone RC, Slotman GJ, Metz CA, Thomas FO, The Methyl-prednisolone Severe Sepsis Study Group (1992) Hypothermia in the sepsis syndrome and clinical outcome. Crit Care Med 20:1395–1401

44. Colman RW (1994) Disseminated intravascular coagulation due to sepsis. Semin Hematol 31 [Suppl 1]:10–17

45. Conary JT, Parker RE, Christman BW, Faulks RD, King GA, Meyrick BO, Brigham KL (1994) Protection of rabbit lungs from endotoxin injury by in vivo hyperexpression of the prostaglandin G/H synthase gene. J Clin Invest 93:1834–1840

46. Conway EM, Rosenberg RD (1988) Tumor necrosis factor suppresses transcription of the thrombomodulin gene in endothelial cells. Mol Cell Biol 8:5588–5592

47. Craven DE (1992) Use of selective decontamination of the digestive tract – Is the light at the end of the tunnel red or green? Ann Intern Med 117:609–611

48. Daly JM, Lieberman MD, Goldfine J, Shou J, Weintraub F, Rosato EF, Lavin P (1992) Enteral nutrition with supplemental arginine, RNA, and omega-3 fatty acids in patients after operation: immunologic, metabolic, and clinical outcome. Surgery 112:56–67

49. Damas P, Ledoux D, Nys M, Vrindts Y, de Groote D, Franchimont P, Lamy M (1992) Cytokine serum level during severe sepsis in human IL-6 as a marker of severity. Ann Surg 215:356–362

50. Desjars P, Pinaud M, Potel G, Tasseau F, Touze MD (1987) A reappraisal of norepi-nephrine therapy in human septic shock. Crit Care Med 15:134–137

51. Dhainaut JFA, Tenaillon A, Le Tulzo Y, Schlemmer B, Solet JP, Wolff M, Holzapfel L, Zeni F, Dreyfuss D, Mira JP, De Vathaire F, Guinot P, the BN 52021 Sepsis Study Group (1994) Platelet-activating factor receptor antagonist BN 52021 in the treatment of severe sepsis: A randomized, double-blind, placebo-controlled, multicenter clinical trial. Crit Care Med 22:1720–1728

52. Dickneite G, Pâques EP (1993) Protection of DIC-induced mortality in Klebsiella peneumoniae-infected and LPS-treated rats by antithrombin III. In: Müller-Berghaus G, Madlener K, Blombäck M, ten Cate JW (eds) DIC: Pathogenesis, Diagnosis and Therapy of Disseminated Intravascular Fibrin Formation. Excerpta Medica, Amsterdam, pp 215–219

53. Dofferhoff AS, de Jong HJ, Bom VJ, van der Meer J, Limburg PC, de Vries-Hospers HG, Marrink J, Mulder PO, Weits J (1992) Complement activation and the production of inflammatory mediators during the treatment of severe sepsis in humans. Scand J Infect Dis 24:197–204

54. Dominioni L, Diongi R, Zanello M, Monico R, Cremaschi R, Diongi R, Ballabio A, Massa M, Comelli M, dal Ri P, Pisati P (1987) Sepsis score and acute-phase protein response as predictors of outcome in septic surgical patients. Arch Surg 122:141–146
55. Dominioni L, Dionigi R, Zanello M, Chiaranda M, Diongi R, Acquarolo A, Ballabio A, Sguotti C (1991) Effects of high-dose IgG on survival of surgical patients with sepsis scores of 20 or greater. Arch Surg 126:236–240
56. Drake TA, Cheng J, Chang A, Taylor FB (1993) Expression of tissue factor, thrombomodulin, and E-selectin in baboons with lethal Escherichia-coli sepsis. Am J Pathol 142:1458–1470
57. Edgington TS, Mackman N, Fan ST, Ruf W (1992) Cellular immune and cytokine pathways resulting in tissue factor expression and relevance to septic shock. Nouv Rev Fr Haematol 34 [Suppl]:S15–S27
58. Elebute EA, Stoner HB (1983) The grading of sepsis. Br J Surg 70:29–31
59. Emerson TE, Fournel MA, Redens TB, Taylor FB (1989) Efficacy of antithrombin III supplementation in animal models of fulminant Escherichia coli endotoxemia or bacteremia. Am J Med 87 (3B):27S–33S
60. Ferrari-Baliviera E, Mealy K, Smith RI, Wilmore DW (1989) Tumor necrosis factor induces adult respiratory distress syndrome in rats. Arch Surg 124:1400–1405
61. Filz HP, Förster H (1994) Sepsis nach Splenektomie – das OPSI-Syndrom. Intensivmedizin 31:288–290
62. Fink MP (1992) Selective digestive decontamination: A gut issue for the nineties [editorial]. Crit Care Med 20:559–562
63. Fisher CJ, Dhainaut JF, Opal SM, Pribble JP, Balk RA, Slotman GJ, Iberti TJ, Rackow EC, Shapiro MJ, Greenman RL, Reines HD et al (1994) Recombinant human interleukin 1 receptor antagonist in the treatment of patients with sepsis syndrome. Results from a randomized, double-blind, placebo-controlled trial. JAMA 271:1836–1843
64. Fisher CJ, Marra MN, Palardy JE, Marchbanks CR, Scott RW, Opal SM (1994) Human neutrophil bactericidal/permeability-increasing protein reduces mortality rate from endotoxin challenge: A placebo-controlled study. Crit Care Med 22:553–558
65. Fletcher JR (1991) Ibuprofen in patients with severe sepsis [editorial]. Crit Care Med 19:1331–1332
66. Fourrier F, Lestavel P, Chopin C, Marey A, Goudemand J, Rime A, Mangalaboyi J (1990) Meningococcemia and purpura fulminans in adults: acute deficiencies of proteins C and S and early treatment with antithrombin III concentrates. Intensive Care Med 16:121–124
67. Fourrier F, Chopin C, Goudemand J, Hendrycx S, Caron C, Rime A, Marey A, Lestavel P (1992) Septic shock, multiple organ failure, and disseminated intravascular coagulation. Compared patterns of antithrombin III, protein C, and protein S deficiencies. Chest 101:816–823
68. Fourrier F, Chopin C, Huart JJ, Runge I, Caron C, Goudemand J (1993) Double-blind, placebo-controlled trial of antithrombin III concentrates in septic shock with disseminated intravascular coagulation. Chest 104:882–888
69. Freund M, Ostendorf P, Gärtner VH, Tidow S (1981) OPSI – Ein Fall foudroyant verlaufender Sepsis. Internist 22:175–179
70. Freye E, Knüfermann V (1994) Keine Hemmung der intestinalen Motilität nach Ketamin/ Midazolamnarkose. Anaesthesist 43:87–91
71. Gastinne H, Wolff M, Delatour F, Faurisson F, Chevret S, French Study Group on Selective Decontamination of the Digestive Tract (1992) A controlled trial in intensive care units of selective decontamination of the digestive tract with nonabsorbable antibiotics. N Engl J Med 326:594–599
72. Gattinoni L, Pesenti A, Bombino M, Baglioni S, Rivolta M, Rossi F, Rossi G, Fumagalli R, Marcolin R, Mascheroni D, Torresin A (1988) Relationships between lung computed tomographic density, gas exchange, and PEEP in acute respiratory failure. Anesthesiology 69:824–832
73. George JN, Shattil SJ (1991) The clinical importance of acquired abnormalities of platelet function. N Engl J Med 324:27–39
74. Glauser MP, Zanetti G, Baumgartner JD, Cohen J (1991) Septic shock: pathogenesis. Lancet 338:732–736

75. Gomez A, Wang R, Unruh H, Light RB, Bose D, Chau T, Correa E, Mink S (1990) Hemofiltration reverses left ventricular dysfunction during sepsis in dogs. Anesthesiology 73:671–685

76. Goode HF, Webster NR (1993) Free radicals and antioxidants in sepsis. Crit Care Med 21:1770–1776

77. Greenman RL, Schein RM, Martin MA, Wenzel RP, MacIntyre NR, Emmanuel G, Chmel H, Kohler RB, McCarthy M, Plouffe J et al (1991) A controlled clinical trial of E5 murine monoclonal IgM antibody to endotoxin in the treatment of gram-negative sepsis. The XOMA Sepsis Study Group. JAMA 266:1097–1102

78. Grootendorst AF, van Bommel EFH, van der Hoven B, van Leengoed LAMG, van Osta ALM (1992) High volume hemofiltration improves right ventricular function in endotoxin-induced shock in the pig. Intensive Care Med 18:235–240

79. Guerrero R, Velasco F, Rodriguez M, Lopez A, Rojas R, Alvarez MA, Villalba R, Rubio V, Torres A, del Castillo D (1993) Endotoxin-induced pulmonary dysfunction is prevented by C1-esterase inhibitor. J Clin Invest 91:2754–2760

80. Hack CE, Voerman HJ, Eisele B, Keinecke HO, Nuijens JH, Eerenberg AJM, Ogilvie A, Schijndel RJMS, van Delvos U, Thijs LG (1992) C1-esterase inhibitor substitution in sepsis [letter]. Lancet 339:378

81. Hack CE, Ogilvie AC, Eisele B, Eerenberg AJM, Wagstaff J, Thijs LG (1993) C1-inhibitor substitution therapy in septic shock and in the vacular leak syndrome induced by high doses of interleukin-2. Intensive Care Med 19:S19–S28

82. Hackshaw KV, Parker GA, Roberts JW (1990) Naloxone in septic shock. Crit Care Med 18:47–51

83. Hammond JMJ, Potgieter PD, Saunders GL, Forder AA (1992) Double-blind study of selective decontamination of the digestive tract in intensive care. Lancet 340:5–9

84. Hardaway RM (1978) Acute respiratory distress syndrome and disseminated intravascular coagulation. South Med J 71:596–598

85. Hardaway RM, Williams CH, Marvasti M, Farias M, Tseng A, Pinon I, Yanez D, Martinez M, Navar J (1990) Prevention of adult respiratory distress syndrome with plasminogen activator in pigs. Crit Care Med 18:1413–1418

86. Hardaway RM, Harke H, Williams CH (1994) Fibrinolytic agents – A new approach to the treatment of adult respiratory distress syndrome. Adv Ther 11:43–51

87. Harke H (1991) Fibrinolysetherapie bei chirurgisch behandelten Intensivpatienten. Klin Wochenschr 69 [Suppl 26]:150–156

88. Hasegawa N, Husari AW, Hart WT, Kandra TG, Raffin TA (1994) Role of the coagulation systems in ARDS. Chest 105:268–277

89. Hayes MA, Timmins AC, Yau EHS, Palazzo M, Hinds CJ, Watson D (1994) Elevation of systemic oxygen delivery in the treatment of critically ill patients. N Engl J Med 330:1717–1722

90. Heard SO, Perkins MW, Fink MP (1992) Tumor necrosis factor- causes myocardial depression in guinea pigs. Crit Care Med 20:523–527

91. High KM, Snider MT, Richard R, Russell GB, Stene JK, Campbell DB, Aufiero TX, Thieme GA (1992) Clinical trials of an intravenous oxygenator in patients with adult respiratory distress syndrome. Anesthesiology 77:856–863

92. Hinshaw LB, Emerson TE, Taylor FB, Chang ACK, Duerr M, Peer GT, Flournoy DJ, White GL, Kosanke SD, Murray CK, Xu R, Passey RB, Fournel MA (1992) Lethal Staphylococcus aureus-induced shock in primates: Prevention of death with ant-TNF antibody. J Trauma 33:568–573

93. Hörmann C, Benzer H, Baum M, Wicke K, Putensen C, Putz G, Hartlieb S (1994) Bauchlagerung im ARDS. Anaesthesist 43:454–462

94. Holaday JW, Faden AI (1978) Naloxone reversal of endotoxin hypotension suggests role of endorphins in shock. Nature 275:450–451

95. Holaday JW, Ruvio BA, Faden AI (1981) Thyrotropin releasing hormone improves blood pressure and survival in endotoxic shock. Eur J Pharmacol 74:101–105

96. Hollenberg SM, Cunnion RE, Parrillo JE (1992) Effect of septic serum on vascular smooth muscle: In vitro studies using rat aortic rings. Crit Care Med 20:993–998

97. Hotchkiss RS, Karl IE (1992) Reevaluation of the role of cellular hypoxia and bioenergetic failure in sepsis. JAMA 267:1503–1510
98. Hudson LD, Milberg JA, Anardi D, Maunder RJ (1995) Clinical risks for development of the acute respiratory distress syndrome. Am J Respir Crit Care Med 151:293–301
99. Idell S, Koenig KB, Fair DS, Martin TR, McLarty J, Maunder RJ (1991) Serial abnormalities of fibrin turnover in evolving adult respiratory distress syndrome. Am J Physiol 261:L240–L248
100. Jackson RJ, Smith SD, Rowe MI (1990) Selective bowel decontamination results in grampositive translocation. J Surg Res 48:444–447
101. Jepsen S, Herlevsen P, Knudsen P, Bud MI, Klausen NO (1992) Antioxidant treatment with N-acetylcysteine during adult respiratory distress syndrome: A prospective, randomized, placebo-controlled study. Crit Care Med 20:918–923
102. Jin H, Yang R, Marsters S, Ashkenazi A, Bunting S, Marra MN, Scott RW, Baker JB (1995) Protection against endotoxic shock by bactericidal/permeability-increasing protein in rats. J Clin Invest 95:1947–1952
103. Jochum M, Inthorn D, Waydhas Ch, Fritz H (1994) Modulation of inflammatory mediators by AT III-therapy [abstract]. Intensive Care Med 20 [Suppl 1]:S119
104. Johnson D, Hurst T, Prasad K, Wilson T, Saxena A, Murphy F, Mayers I (1994) Lazaroid pretreatment preserves gas exchange in endotoxin-treated dogs. J Crit Care 9:213–223
105. Kalter ES, Daha MR, ten Cate JW, Verhoef J, Bouma BN (1985) Activation and inhibition of Hageman factor-dependent pathways and the complement system in uncomplicated bacteremia or bacterial shock. J Infect Dis 151:1019–1027
106. Kirchhofer D, Tschopp TB, Hadvary P, Baumgartner HR (1994) Endothelial cells stimulated with tumor necrosis factor- express varying amounts of tissue factor resulting in inhomogenous fibrin deposition in a native blood flow system. Effects of thrombin inhibitors. J Clin Invest 93:2073–2083
107. Klausner JM, Paterson IS, Goldman G, Kobzik L, Lelzuk S, Skornick Y, Eberlein T, Valeri R, Shepro D, Hechtman HB (1991) Interleukin-2-induced lung injury is mediated by oxygen free radicals. Surgery 109:169–175
108. Knaus WA, Draper EA, Wagner DP, Zimmerman JE (1985) APACHE II: A severity of disease classification system. Crit Care Med 13:818–829
109. Kollef MH, Schuster DP (1995) The acute respiratory distress syndrome. N Engl J Med 332:27–37
110. Koltai M, Hosford D, Braquet P (1992) Role of PAF and cytokines in microvascular tissue injury. J Lab Clin Med 119:461–466
111. Kreimeier U, Meßmer K (1992) Einsatz hypertoner NaCl-Lösungen zur primären Volumentherapie. Zentralbl Chir 117:532–539
112. Kreimeier U, Frey L, Dentz J, Herbel T, Messmer K (1991) Hypertonic saline dextran resuscitation during the initial phase of acute endotoxemia: effect on regional blood flow. Crit Care Med 19:801–809
113. Lasch HG, Heene DH (1975) Heparin therapy of diffuse intravascular coagulation (DIC). Thromb Diath Haemorrh 33:105–106
114. Leclerc F, Hazelzet J, Jude B, Hofhuis W, Hue V, Martinot A, Van der Voort E (1992) Protein C and S deficiency in severe infectious purpura of children: a collaborative study of 40 cases. Intensive Care Med 18:202–205
115. Levi M, ten Cate H, Bauer KA, van der Poll T, Edgington TS, Büller HR, van Deventer SJH, Hack CE, ten Cate JW, Rosenberg RD (1994) Inhibition of endotoxin-induced activation of coagulation and fibrinolysis by pentoxifylline or by a monoclonal anti-tissue factor antibody in chimpanzees. J Clin Invest 93:114–120
116. Lewis JF, Jobe AH (1993) Surfactant and the adult respiratory distress syndrome. Am Rev Respir Dis 147:218–233
117. Liban E, Raz S (1969) A clinicopathologic study of fourteen cases of amniotic fluid embolism. Am J Clin Pathol 51:477–486
118. Lin PJ, Chang CH, Chang JP (1994) Reversal of refractory hypotension in septic shock by inhibitor of nitric oxide synthase. Chest 106:626–629

119. Liu P, Vonderfecht SL, McGuire GM, Fisher MA, Farhood A, Jaeschke H (1994) The 21-aminosteroid tirilazad mesylate protects against endotoxin shock and acute liver failure in rats. J Pharmacol Exp Ther 271:438–445

120. Lorente JA, García-Frade LJ, Landín L, Pablo R de, Torrado C, Renes E, García-Avello A (1993) Time course of hemostatic abnormalities in sepsis and its relation to outcome. Chest 103:1536–1542

121. Lübbe AS, Garrison RN, Cryer HM, Alsip NL, Harris PD (1992) EDRF as a possible mediator of sepsis-induced arteriolar dilation in skeletal muscle. Am J Physiol 262:H880–887

122. Mackman N, Brand K, Edgington TS (1991) Lipopolysaccharide-mediated transcriptional activation of the human tissue factor gene in THP-1 monocytic cells requires both activator protein 1 and nuclear factor B binding sites. J Exp Med 174:1517–1526

123. Mammen EF, Miyakawa T, Phillips TF, Assarian GS, Brown JM, Murano G (1985) Human antithrombin concentrates and experimental disseminated intravascular coagulation. Semin Thromb Hemost 11:373–383

124. Marik PE, Sibbald WJ (1993) Effect of stored-blood transfusion on oxygen delivery in patients with sepsis. JAMA 269:3024–3029

125. Marra MN, Wilde CG, Griffith JE, Snable JL, Scott RW (1990) Bactericidal/permeability-increasing protein has endotoxin-neutralizing activity. J Immunol 144:662–666

126. Marshall JC, Christou NV, Meakins JL (1993) The gastrointestinal tract. The "undrained abscess" of multiple organ failure. Ann Surg 218:111–119

127. Martin C, Saux P, Eon B, Aknin P, Gouin F (1990) Septic shock: a goal-directed therapy using volume loading, dobutamine and/or norepinephrine. Acta Anaesthesiol Scand 34:413–417

128. Mason JW, Kleeberg U, Dolan P, Coleman RW (1970) Plasma kallikrein and Hageman factor in Gram-negative bacteremia. Ann Intern Med 73:545–551

129. McManus ML, Churchwell KB (1993) Coagulopathy as a predictor of outcome in meningococcal sepsis and the systemic inflammatory response syndrome with purpura. Crit Care Med 21:706–711

130. McMullin M, Johnston G (1993) Long term management of patients after splenectomy. Pneumococcal vaccine, lifelong penicillin, and avoidance of protozoal infections [editorial]. Br Med J 307:1372–1373

131. Meadows D, Edwards JD, Wilkins RG, Nightingale P (1988) Reversal of intractable septic shock with norepinephrine therapy. Crit Care Med 16:663–666

132. Meakins JL, Marshall JC (1986) The gastrointestinal tract: The 'motor' of MOF (Panel discussion - multiple-organ-failure syndrome). Arch Surg 121:197–201

133. Michie HR, Manogue KR, Spriggs DR, Revhaug A, O'Dwyer S, Dinarello CA, Cerami A, Wolff SM, Wilmore DW (1988) Detection of circulating tumor necrosis factor after endotoxin administration. N Engl J Med 318:1481–1486

134. Mira JP, Fabre JE, Baigorri F, Coste J, Annat G, Artigas A, Nitenberg G, Dhainaut JFA (1994) Lack of oxygen supply dependency in patients with severe sepsis. A study of oxygen delivery increased by military antishock trouser and dobutamine. Chest 106:1524–1531

135. Mitaka C, Hirata Y, Makita K, Nagura T, Tsunoda Y, Amaha K (1993) Endothelin-1 and atrial natriuretic peptide in septic shock. Am Heart J 126:466–468

136. Moore FA, Feliciano DV, Andrassy RJ, McArdle AH, Booth FV, Morgenstein-Wagner TB, Kellum JM, Welling RE, Moore EE (1992) Early enteral feeding, compared with parenteral, reduces postoperative septic complications. The results of a meta-analysis. Ann Surg 216:172–183

137. Moreau R, Hadengue A, Soupsion T, Kirstetter P, Mamzer MF, Vanjak D, Vauquelin P, Assous M, Sicot C (1992) Septic shock in patients with cirrhosis: Hemodynamic and metabolic characteristics and intensive care unit outcome. Crit Care Med 20:746–750

138. Nast-Kolb, Waydhas Ch, Jochum M, Schweiberer L (1994) Early antithrombin III treatment of patients with severe multiple injuries [abstract]. Intensive Care Med 20 [Suppl 1]: S121

139. Nawroth PP, Stern DM (1986) Modulation of endothelial cell hemostatic properties by tumor necrosis factor. J Exp Med 163:740–745

140. Nürnberger W, Göbel U, Stannigel H, Eisele B, Janssen A, Delvos U (1992) C1-inhibitor concentrate for sepsis-related capillary leak syndrome [letter]. Lancet 339:990
141. Osterud B, Flaegstad T (1983) Increased tissue thromboplastin activity in monocytes of patients with meningococcal infection: related to an unfavourable prognosis. Thromb Haemost 49:5-7
142. Parrillo JE, Burch C, Shelhamer JH, Parker MM, Natanson C, Schuette W (1985) A circulating myocardial depressent substance in humans with septic shock. Septic shock patients with a reduced ejection fraction have a circulating factor that depresses in vitro myocardial cell performance. J Clin Invest 76:1539-1553
143. Patel RT, Deen KI, Youngs D, Warwick J, Keighley RB (1994) Interleukin 6 is a prognostic indicator of outcome in severe intra-abdominal sepsis. Br J Surg 81:1306-1308
144. Petros A, Bennett D, Vallance P (1991) Effect of nitric oxide synthase inhibitors on hypotension in patients with septic shock. Lancet 338:1557-1558
145. Pilz G, Werdan K (1989) Score-Systeme bei Sepsis und septischem Schock: Diagnosestellung, Verlaufsbeurteilung und Therapiekontrolle, Intensivmed 26/Suppl 1:65-71
146. Pilz G, Kreuzer E, Kääb S, Appel R, Werdan K (1994) Early sepsis treatment with immunoglobulins after cardiac surgery in score-identified high-risk patients. Chest 105:76-82
147. Pollack M (1992) Blood exchange and plasmapheresis in sepsis and septic shock [editorial]. Clin Infect Dis 15:431-433
148. Poole GV, Muakkassa FF, Griswold JA (1992) Pneumonia, selective decontamination, and multiple organ failure. Surgery 111:1-3
149. Redens TB, Emerson TE (1989) Antithrombin-III treatment limits disseminated intravascular coagulation in endotoxemia. Circ Shock 28:49-58
150. Redl-Wenzl EM, Armbruster C, Edelmann G, Fischl E, Kolacny M, Wechsler-Fördös A, Sporn P (1990) Noradrenalin im "High Output-low Resistance State" beim septischen Adominalpatienten. Anaesthesist 39:525-529
151. Reinhart K, Spies CD, Meier-Hellmann A, Bredle DL, Hannemann L, Specht M, Schaffartzik W (1995) N-acetylcysteine preserves oxygen consumption and gastric mucosal pH during hyperoxic ventilation. Am J Respir Crit Care Med 151:773-779
152. Reynolds HN, Haupt MT, Thill-Baharozian MC, Carlson RW (1988) Impact of critical care physician staffing on patients with septic shock in a university hospital medical intensive care unit. JAMA 260:3446-3450
153. Ridings PC, Windsor ACJ, Sugerman HJ, Kennedy E, Sholley MM, Blocher CR, Fisher BJ, Fowler AA (1994) Beneficial cardiopulmonary effects of pentoxifylline in experimental sepsis are lost once septic shock is established. Arch Surg 129:1144-1152
154. Rossaint R, Falke KJ, López F, Slama K, Pison U, Zapol WM (1993) Inhaled nitric oxide for the adult respiratory distress syndrome. N Engl J Med 328:399-405
155. Rossaint R, Lewandowski K, Pappert D, Slama K, Falke K (1994) Die Therapie des ARDS. Teil 1: Aktuelle Behandlungsstrategien einschließlich des extrakorporalen Gasaustauschs. Anaesthesist 43:298-308
156. Rossaint R, Pappert D, Gerlach H, Falke K (1994) Die Therapie des ARDS. Teil 2: Neue Behandlungsmethoden - erste klinische Erfahrungen. Anaesthesist 43:364-375
157. Ronco C, Tetta C, Lupi A, Galloni E, Bettini MC, Sereni L, Mariano F, DeMartino A, Montrucchio G, Camussi G, La Greca G (1995) Removal of platelet-activating factor in experimental continuous arteriovenous hemofiltration. Crit Care Med 23:99-107
158. Rothwell PM, Udwadia ZF, Lawler PG (1991) Cortisol response to corticotropin and survival in septic shock. Lancet 337:582-583
159. Royall JA, Berkow RL, Beckman JS, Cunningham MK, Matalon S, Freeman BA (1989) Tumor necrosis factor and interleukin 1 increase vascular endothelial permeability. Am J Physiol 257:L399-L410
160. Ruokonen E, Takala J, Kari A, Alhava E (1991) Septic shock and multiple organ failure, Crit Care Med 19:1146-1151
161. Sánchez-Cantú L, Rode HN, Yun TJ, Christou NV (1991) Tumor necrosis factor alone does not explain the lethal effect of lipopolysaccharide. Arch Surg 126:231-235

162. Saß W, Bergholz M, Seifert J, Hamelmann H (1984) Splenektomie bei Erwachsenen und das OPSI-Syndrom. Dtsch Med Wochenschr 109:1249–1254
163. Sawyer RG, Adams RB, May AK, Rosenlof LK, Pruett TL, Wilmore DW, Dellinger EP, Vangoor H (1993) Antitumor necrosis factor antibody reduces mortality in the presence of antibiotic-induced tumor necrosis factor release. Arch Surg 128:73–78
164. Schedel I, Dreikhausen U, Nentwig B, Höckenschnieder M, Rauthmann D, Balikcioglu S, Coldewey R, Deicher H (1991) Treatment of Gram-negative septic shock with an immunoglobulin preparation: A prospective, randomized clinical trial. Crit Care Med 19:1104–1113
165. Schilling J, Cakmakci M, Bättig U, Geroulanos S (1993) A new approach in the treatment of hypotension in human septic shock by NG-monomethyl-L-arginine, an inhibitor of the nitric oxide synthetase. Intensive Care Med 19:227–231
166. Schneider AJ, Voerman HJ (1991) Abrupt hemodynamic improvement in late septic shock with physiological doses of glucocorticoids [letter]. Intensive Care Med 17:436–437
167. Schumann RR, Leong SR, Flaggs GW, Gray PW, Wright SD, Mathison JC, Tobias PS, Ulevitch RJ (1990) Structure and function of lipopolysaccharide binding protein. Science 249:1429–1431
168. Schuster DP (1995) Fluid management in ARDS: "keep them dry" or does it matter? Intensive Care Med 21:101–103 (Editorial)
169. Schützer KM, Larsson A, Risberg B, Falk A (1993) Lung protein leakage in feline septic shock. Am Rev Respir Dis 147:1380–1385
170. Seitz R, Wolf M, Egbring R, Havemann K (1989) The disturbance of hemostasis in septic shock: role of neutrophil elastase and thrombin, effects of antithrombin III and plasma substitution. Eur J Haematol 43:22–28
171. Semrad SD, Rose ML, Adams JL (1993) Effect of tirilazed mesylate (U74006F) on eicosanoid and tumor necrosis factor generation in healthy and endotoxemic neonatal calves. Circ Shock 40:235–242
172. Shenkar R, Abraham E (1995) Effects of treatment with the 21-aminosteriod, U74389F, on pulmonary cytokine expression following hemorrhage and resuscitation. Crit Care Med 23:132–139
173. Sheth SB, Carvalho AC (1991) Protein S and C alterations in acutely ill patients. Am J Hematol 36:14–19
174. Shoemaker WC, Appel PL, Kram HB, Waxman K, Lee TS (1988) Prospective trial of supranormal values of survivors as therapeutic goals in high-risk surgical patients. Chest 94:1176–1186
175. Shoemaker WC, Appel PL, Kram HB (1992) Role of oxygen debt in the development of organ failure sepsis, and death in high-risk surgical patients. Chest 102:208–215
176. Sibbald WJ, Vincent JL (1995) Roundtable conference on clinical trials for the treatment of sepsis. Brussels, March 12–14, 1994. Chest 107:522–527
177. Siler TM, Swierkosz JE, Hyers TM, Fowler AA, Webster RO (1989) Immunoreactive interleukin-1 in bronchoalveolar lavage fluid of high-risk patients and patients with the adult respiratory distress syndrome. Exp Lung Res 15:881–894
178. Sitrin RG, Brubaker PG, Fantone JC (1987) Tissue fibrin deposition during acute lung injury in rabbits and its relationship to local expression of procoagulant and fibrinolytic activities. Am Rev Respir Dis 135:930–936
179. Smith EF, Kinter LB, Jugus M, Zeid R (1988) Effect of the thrombolytic agent, streptokinase, on the responses to endotoxemia in conscious rats. Circ Shock 25:85–94
180. Snyder F (1990) Platelet-activating factor and related acetylated lipids as potent biologically active cellular mediators. Am J Physiol 259:C697–C708
181. Spies CD, Reinhart K, Witt I, Meier-Hellmann A, Hannemann L, Bredle DL, Schaffartzik W (1994) Influence of N-acetylcysteine on indirect indicators of tissue oxygenation in septic shock patients: Results from a prospective, randomized, double-blind study. Crit Care Med 22:1738–1746
182. Springer TA (1990) Adhesion receptors of the immune system. Nature 346:425–434
183. Stein B, Pfenninger E, Grünert A, Schmitz JE, Hudde M (1990) Influence of continuous haemofiltration on haemodynamics and central blood volume in experimental endotoxic shock. Intensive Care Med 16:494–499

184. Stephens KE, Ishizaka A, Larrick JW, Raffin TA (1988) Tumor necrosis factor causes increased pulmonary permeability and edema. Comparison to septic acute lung injury. Am Rev Respir Dis 137:1364–1370
185. Stevens LE (1983) Gauging the severity of surgical sepsis. Arch Surg 118:1190–1192
186. Stewart TE, Valenza F, Ribeiro SP, Wener AD, Volgyesi G, Mullen JBM, Slutsky AS (1995) Increased nitric oxide in exhaled gas as an early marker of lung inflammation in a model of sepsis. Am J Respir Crit Care Med 151:713–718
187. Stoutenbeek CP, Saene HKF van, Miranda DR, Zandstra DF (1984) The effect of selective decontamination of the digestive tract on colonization and infection rate in multiple trauma patients. Intensive Care Med 10:185–192
188. Suffredini AF, Harpel PC, Parillo JE (1989) Promotion and subsequent inhibition of plasminogen activation after administration of intravenous endotoxin to normal subjects. N Engl J Med 320:1165–1172
189. Suter PM, Suter S, Girardin E, Roux-Lombard P, Grau GE, Dayer JM (1992) High bronchoalveolar levels of tumor necrosis factor and its inhibitors, interleukin-1, interferon, and elastase in patients with adult respiratory distress syndrome after trauma, shock, or sepsis. Am Rev Respir Dis 145:1016–1022
190. Takenaka I, Ogata M, Koga K, Matsumoto T, Shigematsu A (1994) Ketamine suppresses endotoxin-induced tumor necrosis factor alpha production in mice. Anesthesiology 80:402–408
191. Taylor FB, Chang A, Esmon CT, D'Angelo A, Vigano-D'Angelo S, Blick KE (1987) Protein C prevents the coagulopathic and lethal effects of Escherichia coli infusion in the baboon. J Clin Invest 79:918–925
192. Taylor FB, Chang A, Ruf W, Morrissey JH, Hinshaw L, Catlett R, Blick K, Edgington TS (1991) Lethal E. coli septic shock is prevented by blocking tissue factor with monocloncal antibody. Circ Shock 33:127–134
193. The Veterans Administration Systemic Sepsis Cooperative Study Group (1987) Effect of high-dose glucocorticoid therapy on mortality in patients with clinical signs of systemic sepsis. N Engl J Med 317:659–665
194. Thiel M, Bardenheuer HJ (1994) Medikamentöse Therapie der Sepsis. Eine Indikation für Pentoxifyllin? Anaesthesist 43:249–256
195. Tonnesen E, Hansen MB, Höhndorf K, Diamant M, Bendtzen K, Wanscher M, Toft P (1993) Cytokines in plasma and ultrafiltrate during continuous arteriovenous haemofiltration. Anaesth Intens Care 21:752–758
196. Tracey KJ (1991) Tumor necrosis factor (cachectin) in the biology of septic shock syndrome. Circ Shock 35:123–128
197. Tremel H, Kienle B, Weilemann LS, Stehle P, Fürst P (1994) Glutamine dipeptide-supplemented parenteral nutrition maintains intestinal function in the critically ill. Gastroenterology 107:1595–1601
198. Tuchschmidt J, Fried J, Astiz M, Rackow E (1992) Elevation of cardiac output and oxygen delivery improves outcome in septic shock. Chest 102:216–220
199. van der Poll T, Buller HR, ten Cate H, Wortel CH, Bauer KA, van Deventer SJ, Hack CE, Sauerwein HP, Rosenberg RD, ten Cate JW (1990) Activation of coagulation after administration of tumor necrosis factor to normal subjects. N Engl J Med 322:1622–1627
200. van der Poll T, Levi M, Buller HR, van Deventer SJ, de Boer JP, Hack CE, ten Cate JW (1991) Fibrinolytic response to tumor necrosis factor in healthy subjects. J Exp Med 174:729–732
201. van Deventer SJH, Buller HR, ten Cate JW, Aarden LA, Hack CE, Sturk A (1990) Experimental endotoxemia in humans: analysis of cytokine release and coagulation, fibrinolytic, and complement pathways. Blood 76:2520–2526
202. Vinazzer HA (1995) Antithrombin III in shock and disseminated intravascular coagulation. Clin Appl Thrombosis/Hemostasis 1:62–65
203. Vincent JL, Bihari D (1992) Sepsis, severe sepsis or sepsis syndrome: need for clarification [editorial]. Intensive Care Med 18:255–257
204. Vincent JL, Roman A, Backer D de, Kahn RJ (1990) Oxygen uptake/supply dependency. Effects of short-term dobutamine infusion. Am Rev Respir Dis 142:2–7

205. Vincent JL, Bakker J, Marécaux G, Schandene L, Kahn RJ, Dupont E (1992) Administration of anti-TNF antibody improves left ventricular function in septic shock patients. Results of a pilot study. Chest 101:810–815
206. Voerman HJ, Stehouwer CDA, Kamp GJ van, Schindel SRJM van, Groeneveld ABJ, Thijs LG (1992) Plasma endothelin levels are increased during septic shock. Crit Care Med 20:1097–1101
207. Voss R, Matthias FR, Borkowski G, Reitz D (1990) Activation and inhibition of fibrinolysis in septic patients in an internal intensive care unit. Br J Haematol 75:99–105
208. Walmrath D, Schneider T, Pilch J, Grimminger F, Seeger W (1993) Aerosolised prostacyclin in adult respiratory distress syndrome. Lancet 342:961–962
209. Wegener T, Wallin R, Saldeen T (1986) Effect of N-acetylcysteine on fibrin deposition in the rat lung due to intravascular coagulation. Ups J Med Sci 91:45–52
210. Weiss SJ (1989) Tissue destruction by neutrophils. N Engl J Med 300:365–376
211. Werdan K, Boekstegers P, Müller U, Pfeifer A, Pilz G, Reithmann C, Hallström S, Koidl B, Schuster HP, Schlag G (1991) Akute septische Kardiomyopathie: Bestandteil des Multiorganversagens in der Sepsis? Med Klin 86:526–534
212. Wright SD, Ramos RA, Tobias PS, Ulevitch RJ, Mathison JC (1990) CD14, a receptor for complexes of lipopolysaccharide (LPS) and LPS binding protein. Science 249:1431–1433
213. Zabel P, Wolter DT, Schönharting MM, Schade UF (1989) Oxpentifylline in endotoxaemia. Lancet 334:1474–1477
214. Ziegler EJ, Fisher CJ, Sprung CL, Straube RC, Sadoff JC, Foulke GE, Wortel CH, Fink MP, Dellinger RP et al (1991) Treatment of Gram-negative bacteremia and septic shock with HA-1A human monoclonal antibody against endotoxin. A Randomized, double-blind, placebo-controlled trial. N Engl J Med 324:429–436
215. Ziegler TR, Young LS, Benfell K, Scheltinga M, Hortos K, Bye R, Morrow FD, Jacobs DO, Smith RJ, Antin JH et al (1992) Clinical and metabolic efficacy of glutamine-supplemented parenteral nutrition after bone marrow transplantation. A randomized, double-blind, controlled study. Ann Intern Med 116:821–828

CHAPTER 2

Consumption Coagulopathy: Principles of Management

R. Scherer

Summary

In a multiphase process, pathologically increased activity of the plasmatic coagulation pathways leads to an increasing consumption of plasma factors, inhibitors, and platelets. Increased procoagulant activity and platelet activation tend to exhaust the procoagulant potential, leading to an increasing bleeding diathesis. Disseminated fibrin deposition in the microvasculature of the lungs, liver, heart, and kidneys, reactive hyperfibrinolysis, and persistent bleeding can ultimately lead to a systemic collapse of hemostasis with irreversible hypocoagulability.

The therapeutic approach must take into account the phases of progression of the consumption coagulopathy and must aim at restoring the dynamic equilibrium between activators and inhibitors. Especially in trauma, shock, and sepsis, the initial phase of hypercoagulability triggered by procoagulant activation is eventually followed by a progressive decline of global procoagulant factors and inhibitory coagulation parameters. At least by this stage, treatment should include the administration of antithrombin III (AT III) concentrates, dosed according to body weight, to maintain AT III activity at levels above 80% and thus reduce procoagulant turnover. Further dilution of the coagulation potential should be avoided in this hypocoagulable state, so packed red blood cells (RBCs) should be given in conjunction with fresh frozen plasma (FFP), and AT III infusion should continue to maintain plasma activity levels of at least 80%. Procoagulant concentrates such as PPSB should be given only if FFP alone cannot provide sufficiently rapid factor replacement after a rise of inhibitor potential in a patient with a generalized bleeding diathesis.

The Pathophysiology of Disseminated Intravascular Coagulation as a Basis for Three Therapeutic Principles

Multiple organ failure (MOF) is the most common clinically observed preterminal condition in ICU patients who manifest a systemic inflammatory response (SIRS) to a severe primary underlying disease or injury. *Trauma, protracted shock*, and *septic states* are the main conditions that predispose to the generalized (no longer dependent on local demand) activation of various cascade systems such as the complement system, coagulation system, and fibrinolysis [5, 25, 27]. Trauma, shock, and sepsis additionally trigger the activation of leukocytes. In a process analogous to the antigen-antibody-mediated immune response or the inflammatory response, this leukocyte activation triggers the release of mediators ("lymphokines") leading to the procoagulant transformation of endothelial cells and monocytes by the expression of tissue factor (TF) or Mac-1 receptor or the suppression of thrombomodulin [1]. Because the *procoagulant stimulus persists* in these disease states, there is increased pathologic activation and turnover in the coagulation system leading to thrombinemia and disseminated intravascular coagulation (DIC). Widespread fibrin deposition occurring in the microcirculation of the lungs, liver, kidneys, and presumably the brain [14] contributes to tissue ischemia and hypoxia. If subsequent recanalization occurs due to secondary hyperfibrinolysis or therapeutic measures such as volume replacement and arterial pressure elevation, the tissue supplied by the recanalized vessels will be reperfused but will also be subject to additional injury due, for example, to free radical generation by the action of xanthine oxidase ("reperfusion syndrome" [29]).

During this early hypercoagulable phase of DIC, physiologic coagulation inhibitors form complexes with activated coagulation factors that are hemostatically inactive [e.g., thrombin (IIa)-antithrombin III (AT III), factor Xa-AT III], or active coagulation (co)factors are split off (Va and VIIIa by activated protein C and its cofactor protein S), resulting in the progressive consumption of coagulation factors (procoagulants) and coagulation inhibitors The potential exhaustion on the inhibitor side allows the consumption of coagulation factors to proceed unchecked, so that the initial increased turnover in the coagulation system gives rise to a *hypocoagulable state* that is eventually manifested by diffuse bleeding (see Fig. 1). This sequence of events progressing to consumption coagulopathy provides a foundation for defining three basic therapeutic principles:

- Treatment of the underlying cause
- Reduction of procoagulant turnover
- Repletion of inhibitors and procoagulants in the coagulation system

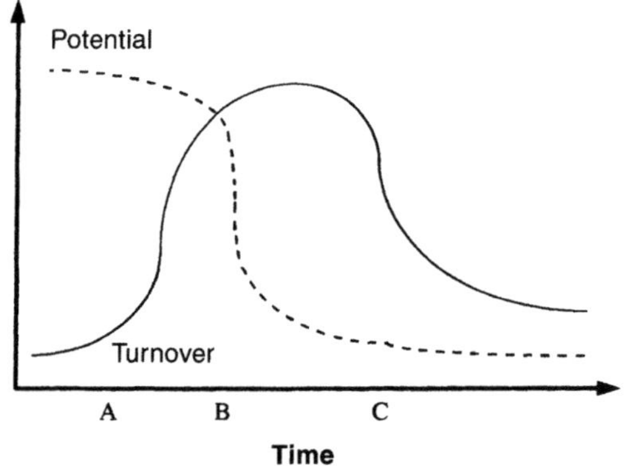

Fig. 1. Progression from initial hypercoagulability to consumption coagulopathy. *Solid line*: coagulation factor turnover; *broken line*: coagulation factor/inhibitor potential. *A* Initial activation of coagulation, with hypercoagulability. *B* Onset of potential decline, marking start of hypocoagulable phase. *C* Potential exhaustion, "burnout" of the consumption coagulopathy

Staged Therapeutic Approach: Capabilities and Limitations of the Treatment of Consumption Coagulopathy with Blood Components

Treatment of the Underlying Cause

Treatment of the condition triggering the pathologic activation of coagulation in sepsis, such as the surgical eradication of a primary infectious focus, is rarely possible. The administration of antibiotics based on sensitivity tests is the measure that most closely approximates causal therapy. But SIRS is associated with the typical hemodynamic pattern of low peripheral vascular resistance, increased capillary permeability, and cardiac function that is initially hyperdynamic and later hypodynamic, much like the findings in shock due to other causes. Consequently, the hemodynamic changes induced by trauma, shock, and sepsis culminate in a common end-state of intravascular hypovolemia and low mean arterial pressure, leading to a reduction of blood flow in the microcirculation (in addition to vascular obstruction by fibrin), which becomes a coagulation-promoting factor.

Multiple trauma and/or hypovolemic-hemorrhagic shock may be followed by the same pathophysiologic changes that lead to a decrease in oxygen delivery to the tissues (DO_2). SIRS, on the other hand, is consistently associated with a pathologic increase in oxygen uptake and demand (VO_2), thereby promoting the development of tissue hypoxia and metabolic acidosis. Hypovolemia, centralization, hypotension, and local hypoxia thus become independent triggers of increased turnover in the coagulation system. Appropriate treatment must include the following measures, therefore.

Adequate Volume Replacement. Volume repletion in severe disease states is guided by invasive measurements of arterial pressure, CVP, mean pulmonary arterial pressure, pulmonary arterial wedge pressure, pulmonary arterial oxygen saturation, and measurement of the cardiac output. It involves the use of crystalline and colloidal infusion solutions or 20% human albumin in hypoalbuminemic patients and the maintenance of a positive fluid balance. The more liberal use of crystalline and colloidal infusion solutions carries a risk of dilutional coagulopathy. Especially with colloidal replacement solutions (e.g., Haes 10%), attention should be given to maximum dose recommendations (1500 ml) due to interference with platelet aggregation and cross matching.

Administration of Catecholamines. Catecholamines help to ensure adequate tissue oxygen delivery by stimulating the cardiac β_2 receptors to maintain a cardiac index greater than 2.5 l min^{-1} m^{-2}. Ordinarily, dopamine is administered first (up to 10 µg kg^{-1} min^{-1}) followed later by epinephrine (initial dose of 0.1 µg kg^{-1} min^{-1}). Patients with an adequate mean arterial pressure (at least 50–60 mm Hg) can also be treated with inodilators with slight peripheral β activity, whose vasodilator properties will improve perfusion (e.g., dobutamine in an initial dose of 3–4 µg kg^{-1} min^{-1}).

Maintenance of Oxygen Delivery by Arterial Blood. The arterial oxygen tension (pO_2) in critically ill patients should exceed 100 mm Hg, and oxygen saturation should exceed 95%. Since patients will generally be on assisted ventilation, this must be accomplished by optimum individual adjustment of the minute ventilation and respiratory rate, the inspiratory-to-expiratory ratio, inspiratory flow, inspiratory pressure limit, and finally the inspired oxygen concentration (F_iO_2).

Reduction of Procoagulant Turnover by Replacing the Inhibitor Potential

The next step consists of inhibiting the pathologic procoagulant activation to reduce the exorbitant turnover of procoagulant factors.

Heparin

Low-dose heparin therapy at 100–150 U/kg/24 h i.v. (roughly equivalent to low-dose prophylaxis) is used in practically all ICU patients and can accelerate response to AT III [8, 17]. Heparin therapy basically requires a normal AT III level of at least 70%. If the inhibitory potential of AT III is accelerated, and thus consumed, by increasing the heparin dose in patients with low AT III levels, the ensuing consumption response can lead to heparinemia or a greater inhibition of coagulation. In these cases it is difficult to calculate the level of AT III replacement needed to restore coagulation inhibition by the heparin-AT III complex, and the administration of AT III can lead to severe hemorrhagic complications. For this reason, higher-dose heparin therapy is contraindicated in patients with activated coagulation and DIC.

Replacement of Antithrombin III

AT III is the most important physiologic inhibitor of the coagulation system. When administered to experimental animals with consumption coagulopathy, usually endotoxin-induced, high doses of AT III can improve survival in all animal species [6, 12, 18, 26, 28]. AT III replacement can normalize the increased turnover of radiolabeled fibrinogen in patients with liver disease [23]. AT III replacement can also reduce thrombin generation in septic patients and patients in prolonged shock with consumption coagulopathy [4, 24]. It is reasonable to assume, then, that AT III replacement can reduce the degree of procoagulant activation and thereby reducing thrombin generation and intravascular fibrin deposition. No studies to date have been able to prove that AT III replacement can significantly increase survival rates in patients with DIC, but studies in this area [2, 4, 7] suggest that this is the case. Thus, the best evidence to date indicates that AT III replacement to plasma activities > 80% in DIC and in sepsis with DIC is the most beneficial of the many supportive therapies in the prevention of multiple organ failure [10].

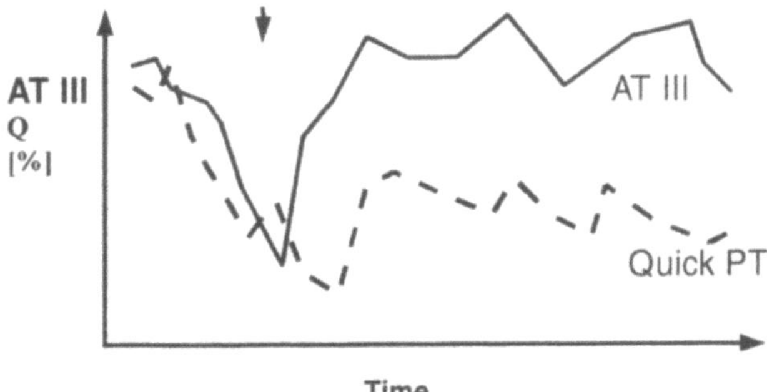

Fig. 2. Principle of AT III replacement. The progressive decline of procoagulants (Quick PT) and inhibitors (AT III) provides the indication for AT III replacement (*arrow*). Procoagulant replacement is indicated only at a later stage

In clinical practice, an AT III assay showing a less than 70% level of AT III activity in itself is not an indication for replacement therapy. In postoperative patients, for example, it is normal to find decreased AT III activity levels along with a reduced procoagulant potential during the initial days following surgery. It is at least necessary to:

- Identify a severe underlying disorder that can trigger the activation of coagulation (e.g., sepsis, peritonitis, multiple trauma, protracted shock). Apparently it is too late for AT III replacement in patients who are already manifesting multiple organ failure. Therefore:
- At the latest, AT III replacement should be initiated in the face of a progressive, consumption-related decline in global procoagulant parameters (PT, Quick PT, TT, fibrinogen, platelet count) and inhibitors (AT III). This AT III replacement should be administered promptly and in an adequate dose. Raising the activity to 80%–100% follows the clinical rule of thumb that 1 U per kg body weight will increase the plasma activity of AT III by approximately 1% [15]. The requisite dose is divided, with 50% administered initially and 50% about 6 h later. Close monitoring of AT III activity is necessary to ensure a good response, since in vivo recovery of the concentrates can vary with the nature of the disease [21]. The plasma AT III level should be constantly maintained at 80%–100% and should be significantly greater than the Quick PT, which also is expressed as a percentage and so is easily compared with the AT III (Fig. 2).

Fresh Frozen Plasma

If an existing bleeding diathesis requires the continuous transfusion of packed RBCs, fresh frozen plasma (FFP) should also be administered as an adjunct. FFP is commonly misused in ICUs and operating suites as a simple volume expander [11]. A 1:1 transfusion of packed RBCs and FFP should be considered:

- Whenever major surgery is performed in patients with a *severe preexisting plasmatic coagulation disorder* (e.g., hepatic cirrhosis)
- In patients who show a *diffuse bleeding diathesis*
- In cases where *surgical bleeding cannot be controlled in a reasonable period of time* [22].

For the future, it should be determined whether quarantine procedures should perhaps be supplemented by the use of virus-inactivated FFP products. Monitoring of the ionized calcium in the plasma is essential in these cases to avoid calcium depletion due to chelation by the excess citrate contained in the blood product.

Replacement of the Procoagulant Potential

Procoagulant concentrates (factor concentrates) should be administered as a third treatment step only after there has been adequate repletion of the inhibitor potential. Factor concentrates should be administered to patients with clinically diffuse bleeding whenever FFP alone cannot significantly improve the PTT and aPTT. This may be the case, for example, when approximately 3000 U would be needed to increase the Quick PT to at least 30%–40% (i.e., with a Quick PT of 5% in a patient weighing 70 kg), requiring an infusion of 3000 ml of FFP (1 ml corresponds to 1 U of each factor and inhibitor). The only indication for giving procoagulant concentrates in the absence of active diffuse bleeding would be a scheduled invasive procedure (central venous catheterization, exploratory surgery) that would necessitate a higher procoagulant potential.

The Prothrombin Complex Concentrate PPSB

The prothrombin complex concentrate PPSB contains factor II (*prothrombin*), factor VII (*proconvertin*), factor X (Stuart-Prower factor), and factor IX (antihemophilic factor *B*). Besides its use in the treatment of vitamin K antagonist overdose, PPSB is administered in liver-related hemostatic defects to effect a rapid repletion of procoagulants in the coagulation system. As with AT III, the requisite dose can be calculated from the current and desired Quick PT and the patient's body weight. Prothrombin complex concentrates also contain proteins C and S [26], providing simultaneous replacement on the inhibitor side. The function of the protein C/S system is particularly impaired in experimental endotoxemia, since both endotoxin [16] and TNF [3] can induce the suppression of thrombomodulin on the endothelial cell surface. Because factor V significantly influences the activity of Xa+Va, Ca^{2+}, and phospholipid complex, the anti-Va and anti-VIIIa actions of protein C cause it to play a key role in the inhibition of prothrombin activation [13]. Other factor concentrates that would be of theoretical benefit in this phase of treatment, such as fibrinogen or factor XIII concentrates, do not have an established indication in DIC. These latter concentrates act at a relatively late stage where only limited potential remains for physiologic inhibition, so there is a risk of increased intravascular fibrin formation in states of pathologically activated coagulation. A general rule governing treatment with procoagulant factor concentrates is that such concentrates should not be used in the absence of a demonstrable factor deficiency, in the absence of clinical diffuse bleeding, and without prior correction of turnover by treatment with antithrombin III.

Platelet Products

Because platelet function tests are not always available for routine clinical use, and bleeding time is not a reliable indicator in critically ill, hemodynamically unstable patients [9], the transfusion of platelet products should be guided by the patient's platelet count and clinical bleeding tendency. Platelet counts lower than 50 000/ μl generally constitute an indication for platelet infusion in the bleeding patient.

Aprotinin should be used with extreme caution in patients who continue to bleed after the previous therapeutic steps have been completed. With reactive hyperfibrinolysis like that typically occurring in DIC, antifibrinolytic agents can promote intravascular fibrin deposition by inhibiting the action of plasmin. Thus, antifibrinolytic agents are mainly indicated for the treatment of primary hyperfibrinolysis (e.g., in obstetrics). If the persistence of diffuse bleeding is referable to a systemically amplified reactive hyperfibrinolysis, a trial of aprotinin may be warranted. In contrast to ε-aminocaproic acid, there is no evidence that aprotinin will exacerbate disseminated fibrin formation in this situation.

References

1. Altieri DC, Morrissey JH, Edgington TS (1988) Adhesive receptor Mac-1 coordinates the activation of factor X on stimulated cells of monocytic and myeloid differentiation: an alternative initiation of the coagulation protease cascade. Proc Natl Acad Sci USA 85:7462–7466
2. Bardenheuer M, Obertacke U, Kleinschmidt C, Scherer R, Eisold C, Jochum M, Schmit-Neuerburg KP (1994) Prophylactic continuous application of antithrombin III (140% serum activity for 4 days after trauma) for reduction of shock related complications and pulmonary microvascular permeability - a prospective clinical study. Am J Resp Crit Care Med 149:A368
3. Bevilacqua MP, Pober JS, Majeau GR, Fiers W, Cotran RS, Gimbrone MA (1986) Recombinant tumor necrosis factor induces procoagulant activity in cultured human vascular endothelium: characterization and comparison with the actions of interleukin 1. Proc Natl Acad Sci USA 83:4533–4537
4. Blauhut B, Kramar H, Vinazzer H, Bergmann H (1985) Substitution of antithrombin III in shock and DIC: a randomised study. Thromb Res 39:81–89
5. Bone RC (1992) mondulators of coagulation. A critical appraisal of their role in sepsis. Arch Intern Med 152:1381–1389
6. Dickneite G, Pâques EP (1993) Reduction of mortality with antithrombin III in septicemic rats: a study of Klebsielle pneumoniae induced sepsis. Thromb Haemostas 69:98–102

7. Fourrier F, Chopin C, Huart JJ, Runge I, Caron C, Goudemand J (1993) Double blind, placebo controlled trial of antithrombin III concentrates in septic shock with disseminated intravascular coagulation. Chest 104:882–888

8. Himmelreich G, Riess H (1993) Pathophysiologie und Therapie der Verbrauchskoagulopathie. Klin Lab 39:25–30

9. Hougie C (1991) Bleeding time. In: Williams WJ, Beutler E, Erslev AJ, Lichtman MA (eds) Hematology. McGraw Hill, New York, pp 1775–1776

10. Kienast J, Ostermann H, Mesters R (1994) Gerinnungsinhibitoren bei Sepsis und disseminierter intravasaler Gerinnung. In: Martin E, Nawroth P (Hrsg.) Fachübergreifende Aspekte der Hämostaseologie. Springer, Berlin Heidelberg New York Tokyo, S 19–36

11. Kretschmer V (1990) Perioperative Gerinnungstherapie und -diagnostik. Infusionstherapie 17 [Suppl]:9–19

12. Mammen EF, Miyakawa T, Phillips TF, Assarian GS, Brown JM, Murano G (1985) Human antithrombin concentrates and experimental disseminated intravascular coagulation. Semin Thromb Hemost 11:373–383

13. Mann KG (1984) Membrane-bound enzyme complexes in blood coagulation. In: Spaet TH (ed) Progress in hemostasis and thrombosis. Grune & Stratton, New York, pp 1–23

14. McKay DG, Margaretten W, Csavossy I (1966) An electron microscope study of the effects of bacterial endotoxin on the blood vascular system. J Lab Invest 15:1815–1829

15. Menitove JE (1991) Preparation and clinical use of plasma and plasma fractions. In: Williams WJ, Beutler E, Erslev AJ, Lichtman MA (eds) Hematology. McGraw Hill, New York, pp 659–673

16. Moore KL, Andreoli SP, Esmon NL, Esmon CT, Bang NU (1987) Endotoxin enhances tissue factor and suppresses thrombomodulin expression of human vascular endothelium in vitro. J Clin Invest 79:124–130

17. Paar D (1991) Diagnostik und Therapie von Hämostasestörungen in der Intensivmedizin. In: Luboldt W, Maurer C (Hrsg.) Entwicklungen in der Transfusionsmedizin. Ecomed, Landsberg am Lech, S 27–33

18. Redens TB, Leach WJ, Bogdanoff DA, Emerson TE (1988) Synergistic protection from lung damage by combining antithrombin III and alpha 1-proteinase inhibitor in the E. coli endotoxemic sheep pulmonary dysfunction model. Circ Shock 26:15–26

19. Riess H, Binsack T, Hiller E (1985) protein C antigen in prothrombin complex concentrates: content, recovery, and half life. Blut 50:303–306

20. Scherer R, Bredendiek M, Paar D, Luboldt W (1991) Komponententherapie und Hämostase bei orthotoper Lebertransplantation. In: Luboldt W, Maurer C (Hrg) Entwicklungen in der Transfusionsmedizin. Ecomed, Landsberg am lech, S 27–33

21. Scherer R, Gödde S, Giebler R, Schmutzler M, Erhard J, Kox WJ (1993) Recovery of antithrombin III in patients undergoing orthotopic liver transplantation after administration of an antithrombin III concentrate, Semin Thromb Hemost 19:309–310

22. Scherer R, Paar D, Stöcker L, Kox WJ (1994) Diagnose und Therapie pathologischer Gerinnungsaktivierungen. Anästhesist 43: 347–354

23. Schipper HG, Ten Cate JW (1982) Antithrombin III transfusion in patients with hepatic cirrhosis. Br J Haematol 52:25–33

24. Seitz R, Wolf M, Egbring R, Havemann VK (1989) The disturbance of hemostasis in septic shock: Role of neutrophile elastase and thrombin, effects of antithrombin III and plasma substitution. Eur J Haematol 43:22–28

25. Tanaka T, Tsujinaka T, Kambayashi J, Higashiyama M, Sakon M, Mori T (1989) Sepsis model with reproducible manifestations of multiple organ failure (MOF) and disseminated intravascular coagulation (DIC). Thromb Res 54:53–61

26. Taylor FB, Emerson TE, Jordan R, Chang AK, Blick KE (1988) Antithrombin III prevents the lethal effects of Escherichia coli infusion in baboons. Circ Shock 26:227–235

27. Thijs LG, Boer JP de, Groot MCM de, Hack CE (1993) Coagulation disorders in septic shock. Intensive Care Med 19:S8–S15

28. Triantaphyllopoulos DC (1984) Effects of human antithrombin III on mortality and blood coagulation induced in rabbits by endotoxin. Thromb Haemostas 51:232–235

29. Ward PA, Mulligan MS, Warren JS (1993) Neutrophils, cytokines, oxygen radicals, and lung injury. In: Faist E, Meakins J, Schildberg FW (eds) Host defense dysfunction trauma, shock and sepsis. Springer, Berlin Heidelberg New York Tokyo, pp 177–180

Part II

Acquired Inhibitors

CHAPTER 3

Acquired Inhibitors Against Factor VIII and Factor IX

I. Scharrer

Summary

Patients with spontaneously acquired factor VIII and factor IX inhibitors generally have a severe, diffuse bleeding diathesis. These inhibitors occur with equal frequency in men and women and are most common in the ranges of 20–30 and 60–80 years of age. The hemorrhagic diathesis is usually manifested by cutaneous and muscular bleeding, intra- and postoperative bleeding, and intraabdominal hemorrhage. Hemarthrosis is far less common than in patients with therapy-induced isoantibodies. The underlying disease may be an autoimmune disorder or a solid neoplasm. Postpartum inhibitors and drug-induced autoantibodies are usually transient but may cause a severe bleeding diathesis. Diagnosis starts with the PTT, and abnormal mixing tests in the PTT screen can suggest the presence of an inhibitor-associated hemorrhagic disorder. The diagnosis is established by the Bethesda assay. The autoantibodies are distinguished from the therapy-induced inhibitors in hemophilia by their complex kinetics. The mortality rate is very high, ranging from 20% to 30%. The first treatment priority is the control of bleeding. This can be accomplished with activated PCC (Feiba), porcine factor VIII (Hyate C), or recombinant factor VIIa. Experimental therapies for antibody elimination involve the use of γ-globulins and/or immunosuppressant therapy.

Acquired antibodies against coagulation factors can occur in healthy individuals as well as in patients with underlying diseases. As a rule, spontaneously acquired inhibitors to factors VIII and IX are associated with severe, life-threatening hemorrhage. The autoantibodies differ from the therapeutically induced isoantibodies in hemophilia both in their kinetics and in their clinical manifestations.

Case Descriptions

We present the following three case descriptions to illustrate the clinical importance of spontaneously acquired factor VIII and IX inhibitors:

A 70-year-old woman who had undergone radiotherapy for cervical carcinoma was admitted with massive uterine bleeding and extensive musculocutaneous bleeding about the hip and thigh (Fig. 1). Her hemoglobin level had fallen to 5 g%. Coagulation studies were abnormal: PTT was prolonged to 72 s, the factor VIII level was 10%, and the inhibitor titer was 20 Bethesda U.

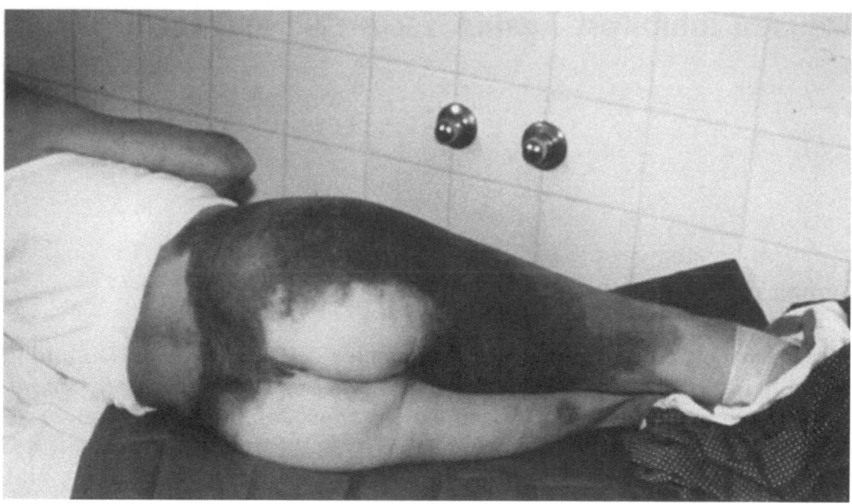

Fig. 1. Extensive musculocutaneous bleeding in a patient with factor VIII inhibitors

A healthy 59-year-old man complained suddenly of dizziness and severe headache. He lost consciousness within 6 h. He had no history of hypertension, and none was measured on admission. CT disclosed a cerebral hemorrhage (Fig. 2). The hemoglobin level was 12.5 g%. Coagulation studies showed abnormal prolongation of PTT to 80 s, a factor VIII level of 8%, and an inhibitor titer of 15 Bethesda U with otherwise normal coagulation parameters. Unfortunately, the patient did not survive the hemorrhage. The source of the inhibitor was not discovered.

The third case illustrates the life-threatening potential of a postpartum inhibitor in a 26-year-old woman. While delivering her first child, the patient

Fig. 2. CT scan of cerebral hemorrhage

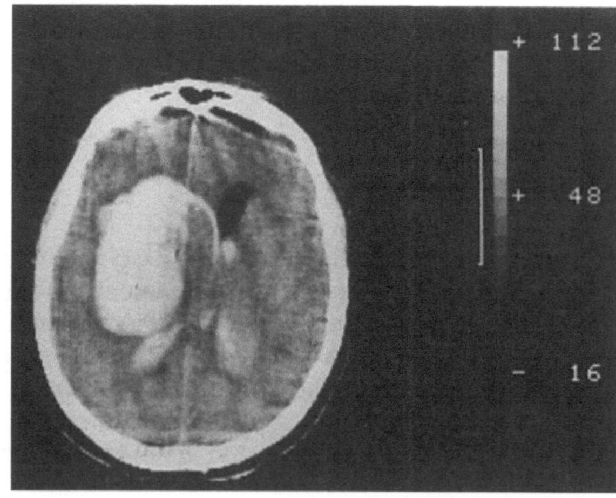

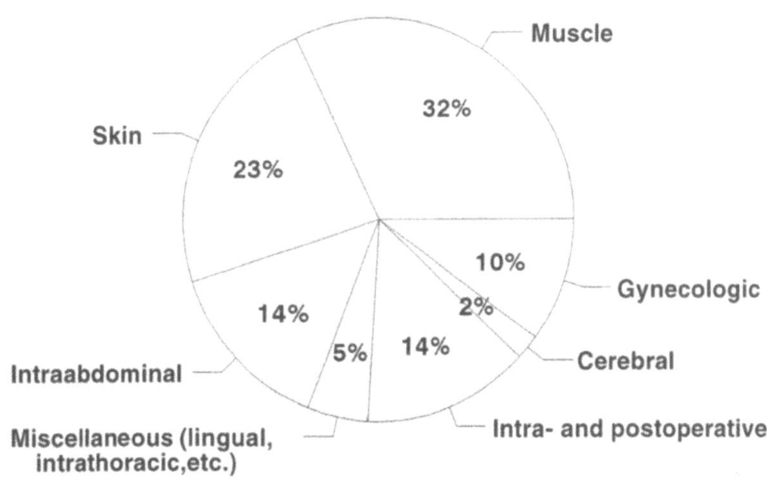

Fig. 3. Bleeding diathesis in patients with "spontaneously acquired" inhibitors

suffered massive uterine bleeding that persisted during the postpartum period. Her hemoglobin level fell to 4.5 g%, and the patient went into shock. Hysterectomy was performed to establish hemostasis. When massive bleeding continued postoperatively, the patient was transferred to our unit. The hemoglobin level on admission was 4.5 g%, PTT was prolonged to 100 s, the factor VIII level had fallen to 5%, and the inhibitor titer was 40 Bethesda U. The infant was found to have a cerebral hemorrhage and showed a factor VIII level of 20% and an inhibitor titer of 10 Bethesda U.

These clinical examples illustrate three typical features of acquired factor inhibitors:

- A severe, diffuse bleeding diathesis
- An equal prevalence in men and women
- A biphasic age distribution with a peak occurrence in the ranges of 20–30 and 60–80 years

Location of Bleeding Sites and Underlying Causes

In contrast to congenital hemophilia, hemarthrosis is very rare in patients with acquired factor inhibitors. The massive bleeding diathesis leads to a very high mortality, with Green and Lechner [9] reporting a 22% death rate in 215 nonhemophilic patients with factor VIII inhibitors. The distribution of bleeding tendencies among our patients, shown in Fig. 3, is consistent with published data. Muscular and cutaneous bleeding are predominant, followed by intra- and postoperative bleeding and intraabdominal hemorrhage.

An underlying disease cannot always be demonstrated. As Fig. 4 shows, factor VIII inhibitors are classified as idiopathic in more than 50% of cases. Green and Lechner [9] found a 46.1% incidence of idiopathic cases. Auto-

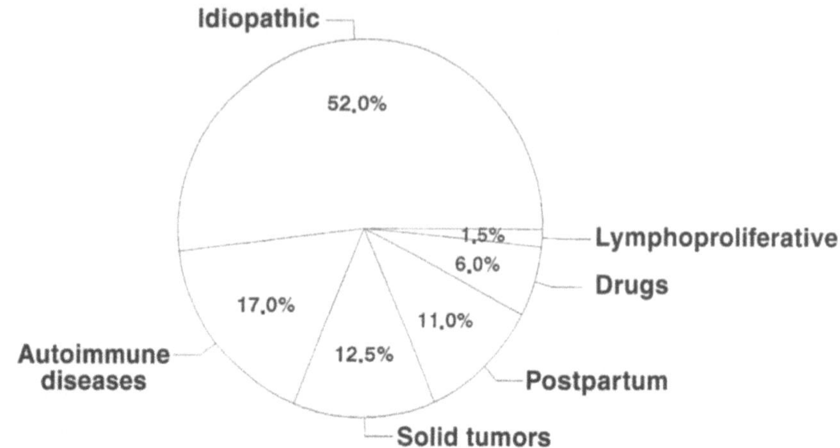

Fig. 4. Underlying diseases in patients with "spontaneously acquired" inhibitors

immune disorders and solid tumors are frequently identified as causes [1, 14, 18, 24]. Postpartum inhibitors [2, 6, 10, 19, 20, 22, 26] are usually detected during or after delivery; prenatal bleeding is very rare. The precise time at which postpartum inhibitors develop is unclear [12, 13]. A review of the literature by Coller et al. [4] indicates that there is no significant risk of inhibitor recurrence during subsequent pregnancies. Drugs that can induce factor VIII inhibitors include ciprofloxacin [3], penicillin, ampicillin, chloramphenicol, nitrofuradantine, and phenytoin [25]. These factor VIII inhibitors are usually transient but can still cause a severe bleeding diathesis.

Laboratory Diagnosis

Diagnosis starts with a PTT screening test. Abnormal mixing results in the test can initially suggest the presence of an inhibitor [25]. Once suspicion has been raised, a specific factor analysis should follow. Factor activity can be determined with the Bethesda assay [15]. The reaction between factor VIII and the inhibitor depends on the temperature and incubation time. An optimum reaction is obtained in samples incubated at 37°C for 2 h.

One Bethesda unit is defined as the concentration that neutralizes 50% of added factor VIII in a mixture incubated at 37°C for 2 h [7, 29]. The percentage of residual factor VIII activity (ordinate) plotted against the inhibitor units (abscissa) produces a characteristic straight line (Fig. 5).

The affinity of the inhibitor for factor VIII is variable. As a general rule, residual factor VIII activity can still be measured in patients with a spontaneously acquired inhibitor. A complex type II kinetic pattern is usually present. This marks a significant difference between acquired inhibitors and the isoantibodies in hemophilia. With hemophilic isoantibodies, the inhibitor is completely saturated in a process with simple type I kinetics, and it displays a

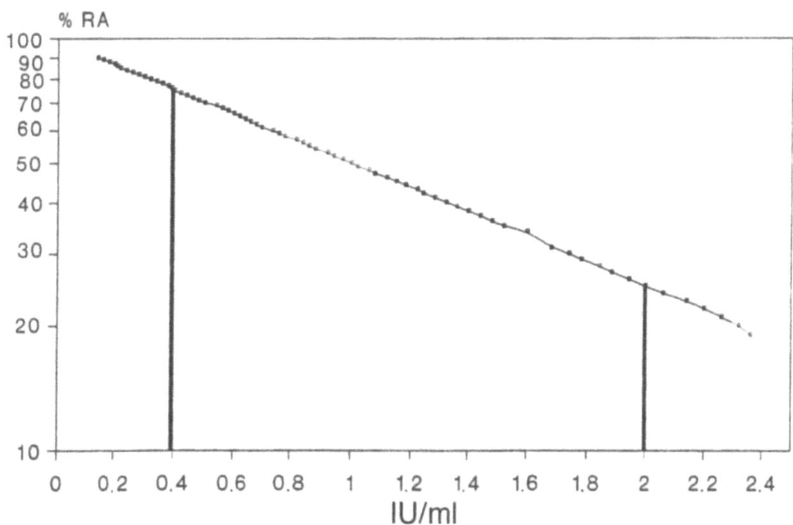

Fig. 5. Bethesda assay (residual activity plotted against inhibitor units)

high affinity for factor VIII. Thus, inhibitor titers can be measured more precisely in immune-inhibitor hemophilia than in patients with auto-antibodies. As a rule, five dilutions must be prepared in order to determine an inhibitor with complex kinetics. The inhibitor titer rises in the laboratory sample, so it is best to state the titer corresponding to a residual activity of 50%.

The inhibitor neutralizes only factor VIII coagulant (VIII:C), not the von Willebrand factor. The autoantibody may be directed against both the heavy chain and the light chain of VIII:C. Factor VIII:C is composed of a heavy chain with the epitopes A1, A2, the B domain, and a light chain with the epitopes A3 and C1/C2, to which the von Willebrand factor is bound. In terms of the epitopes against which the factor VIII inhibitors are directed, no differences have been found between patients with spontaneous inhibitors and those with hemophilic inhibitors following treatment with plasma preparations and re-combinant factor VIII products. The inhibitors act mainly on the A2 and C2 epitopes.

Structurally, autoantibodies are mostly immunoglobulins of the IgG$_1$ to IgG$_4$ subtypes with k and l chains. IgM and IgA inhibitors are rare. Unfortunately, protein A Sepharose is not effective for the removal of inhibitors belonging to the IgG$_3$ subtype.

Therapeutic Approach

The treatment of autoantibodies is a long, arduous, and costly process both in the control of emergency bleeding and in the elimination of factor VIII inhibitors. Emergency treatment can include the use of porcine factor VIII (Hyate C), recombinant factor VIIa, and Feiba.

Spontaneously acquired inhibitors have a lower affinity for porcine factor VIII than for human factor VIII. Before porcine factor VIII is used, cross-reactivity should be tested to determine the relation of the inhibitor against Hyate C to the inhibitor against human factor VIII. If it is greater than 35%, treatment with Hyate C generally will not be effective. Anamnestic titer elevations following the use of Hyate C are very rare. There is no risk of transmission of HIV or hepatitis virus [16]. The dosage is 50–100 U administered twice daily. Thrombocytopenia may occur as a side effect, depending on the dose. Corticosteroids should be given before each infusion due to the potential for an allergic response.

Recombinant factor VIIa can also be used for emergency hemostasis, but currently it is available from Novo Nordisk only for study purposes. It is injected, not infused, in a dose of 90 μg/kg body weight at 2-h intervals, and usually only two or three applications are needed to achieve hemostasis. An anamnestic response (titer elevation) does not occur after use [5, 27].

Feiba, an activated prothrombin complex concentrate (PCC), can also be used for hemostasis. Doses higher than 200 U/kg body weight/day are contraindicated due to the risk of inciting a consumption coagulopathy. An anamnestic response may follow the administration of Feiba in rare instances. Most experience in Germany has been with the use of this activated product.

The inhibitor titer can be lowered by means of plasmapheresis, which can reduce titers by 30%–50% per separation [11]. The usual regimen is to exchange 3 l per day for 5 days with albumin replacement. We successfully used adsorption plasmapheresis in four patients with factor VIII inhibitors using tryptophan polyvinyl alcohol adsorption columns [21]. Figure 6 shows the course of PTT, inhibitors, and factor VIII in one patient who was successfully treated by Mondorf using adsorption plasmapheresis. In the protein A Sepharose technique, known also as the Malmö protocol [23], the protein A Sepharose column is supplemented by combined treatment with intravenous IgG, cyclophosphamide, and factor VIII. Knöbel et al. [17] successfully used IgA apheresis with Therasorb columns in two patients with spontaneous factor VIII inhibitors. One session lasts only 4 h, during which 4–6 l of plasma can be processed.

Attempts have been made to eliminate autoantibodies by treatment with γ-globulins and/or immunosuppressant therapy. γ-Globulins are administered in a daily dose of 0.4 g/kg body weight for 5 days. Studies by Sultan et al. [28] indicate that the presence of anti-idiotype antibodies is responsible for the efficacy of this therapy. It has been our experience that the combination of intravenous immunoglobulin (IVIG) with corticosteroids (1–2 mg/kg body weight) and cyclophosphamide (200 mg/day for 8 days) is more effective than IVIG alone.

Azathioprine, vincristine, cyclosporin A, and interferon α have also been used for the immunosuppression of factor VIII [8].

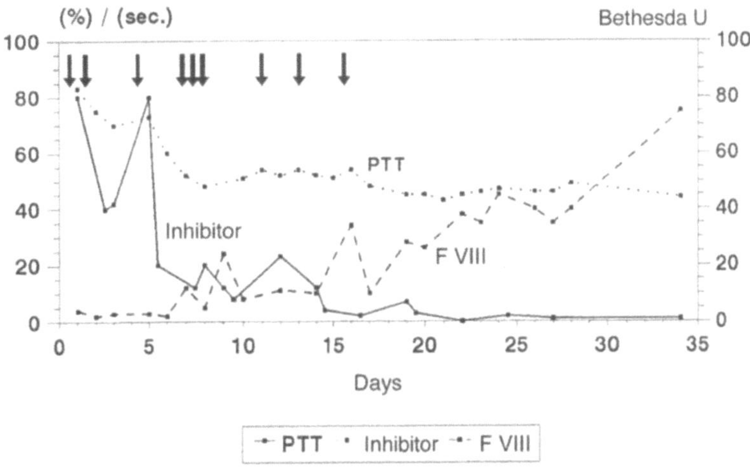

Fig. 6. Course of factor VIII inhibitor and PTT during adsorption plasmapheresis (Immunosorba column)

Acquired Factor IX Inhibitors

Spontaneously acquired factor IX inhibitors are far less common than factor VIII inhibitors. The underlying disorders and bleeding diathesis are similar to those in patients with spontaneous factor VIII inhibitors. Known underlying conditions include malignant tumors and postpartum states. Drug-induced factor IX inhibitors have also been observed following antibiotic use. In their biochemical structure, factor IX inhibitors also belong to the class of IgG antibodies. Unlike factor VIII autoantibodies, they usually show simple type I kinetics, so spontaneous factor IX inhibitors can be more accurately determined by the Bethesda assay. Recombinant factor VIIa and Feiba can be used in the emergency treatment of hemorrhagic episodes. γ-Globulins, cyclophosphamide, and corticosteroids have been successfully used for the elimination of factor IX inhibitors.

Prognosis

The prognosis of spontaneously acquired factor VIII or factor IX inhibitors depends largely on the success of immediate hemostasis in the face of an often life-threatening diffuse bleeding diathesis. With considerable effort, this can be accomplished in approximately 70% of patients. Elimination therapy is successful in about 50% of cases. Spontaneous remissions generally occur only in patients with postpartum and/or drug-induced inhibitors.

In a literature survey by Hauser et al. [13] on the use of postpartum factor VIII inhibitors, it was found that immunosuppressants such as cyclophosphamide and azathioprine greatly shorten the time to complete remission, but that this is not accomplished with the use of corticosteroids alone. Since these patients are frequently at risk for massive bleeding, as our third case illustrates, immediate treatment is still required even if there is a good chance that remission will occur within a period of months or years.

References

1. Al-Ismail SAD, Parry DH, Moisey CU, Bloom AL (1979) Factor VIII inhibitor and bronchogenic carcinoma. Thromb Haemost 41:291
2. Amamiya A, Hamada H, Yamada K, Meguro T (1982) A case of woman with acquired factor VIII inhibitor after the delivery. Rinsho Ketsueki 23:658–665
3. Beek EJR van, Peters M, ten Cate JW (1993) Factor VIII inhibitor associated with ciprofloxacin. Thromb Haemost 69:403
4. Coller BS, Hultin MB, Hoyer LW, Miller F, Dobbs JV, Dosik MH, Berger ER (1981) Normal Pregnancy in a Patient With a prior Postpartum Factor VIII Inhibitor: With Observations on Pathogenesis and Prognosis. Blood 58 3:619–624
5. Doughty HA, Northeast A, Sklair L, Roques T, Young AE, Savidge GF, Hunt BJ (1995) The use of recombinant factor VIIa in a patient with acquired haemophilia A undergoing surgery. Blood Coagulat Fibrinol 6:125–128
6. Files JC, Morrison FS, Halbrook J (1981) Post-partum treatment of a patient with a factor FVIII inhibitor. N Engl J Med 1650
7. Goldsmith JC (1993) Diagnosis of Factor VIII Versus Nonspecific Inhibitors. Semin Hematol 30 2 [Suppl 1]:3–6
8. Green D (1993) Immunosuppression of Factor VIII Inhibitors in Nonhemophilic Patients. Semin Hematol 30/2 [Suppl 1]:28–31
9. Green D, Lechner KA (1981) A survey of 214 nonhemophilic patients with inhibitors to factor VIII. Thromb Haemost 45:200
10. Haedicke G, O'Sullivan J, Seidler C, Donat, Crowley JP (1990) Tracheal obstruction after emergency tracheostomy in a patient with a postpartum factor VIII inhibitor. Crit Care Med 18:449–450
11. Hambley H, Watkins R, Tansey PA, Walker ID, Davidson JF (1985) Plasmapheresis and Factor VIIIC Inhibitors. Lancet n:274
12. Hauser I, Gisslinger H, Locker G, Elbl W, Kyrle PA, Pabinger I, Lechner K (1993) Postpartum factor III inhibitors. Wien Klin Wochenschr 105:355–458
13. Hauser I, Schneider B, Lechner K (1995) Post-Partum Factor VIII Inhibitors. Thromb Haemost 73 1:1–5
14. Hultin MB (1991) Acquired inhibitors in malignant and nonmalignant disease states. Am J Med 91 [Suppl 5 A]:13S
15. Kasper CK, Aledort LM, Counts RB (1975) A more uniform measurement of factor VIII inhibitors. Thromb Diath Haemorrh 34:869–872
16. Kessler CM, Ludlam CA (1993) for the International Acquired Hemophilia Study Group: The Treatment of Acquired Factor VIII Inhibitors: Worldwide Experience With Porcine Factor VIII concentrate. Semin Hematol 30/2 [Suppl 1]:22–27
17. Knöbl P, Derfler K, Korninger L, Jäger U, Maier-Dobersberger T, Druml W, Pabinger I, Lechner K (1995) Elimination of acquired factor VIII inhibitors with immunglobuline-apheresis. Poster no 143, GTH, 15.-18. 2. 1995, Berlin, Ann Hematol 70 [Suppl I]:A36
18. Lionnet F, Pulik M, Genet P, Lucas G, Sollet JP (1995) Acquired factor VIII inhibitor associated with a prostatic cancer: Simultaneous occurrence and healing. Thromb Haemost 73 2:327–328
19. Lutze G, Canzler E, Presser HJ (1989) Spontaner Gerinnungsfaktor-VIII: C-Inhibitor postpartum – Ursache lebensbedrohlicher Blutung. Zentralbl Gynaekol 111:67–172
20. Michiels JJ, Bosch LJ, van der Plas PM, Abels J (1978) Factor VIII inhibitor postpartum. Scand J Haematol 20:7–107
21. Mondorf W, Grützmacher P, Schmidt H, Wolff B, Scharrer I, Baum H von, Hunstein W (1990) Adsorptionsplasmapherese – eine neue Therapiemöglichkeit für Faktor VIII-In-

hibitoren. In: Landbeck G, Marx R, Scharrer I, Schramm W (Hrsg) 20. Hämophilie-Symposion Hamburg 1989. Springer, Heidelberg New York Tokyo, S 345–354
22. Neidhardt B, Bartels O, Hahn B (1985) Hemmkörperhämophilie A postpartum. Dtsch Med Wochenschr 110:799–802
23. Nilsson IM, Berntorp E, Zettervall O (1981) Induction of immune tolerance in patients with hemophilia and antibodies to factor VIII by combined treatment with intravenous IgG, cyclophosphamide and factor VIII. N Engl J Med 15:947–950
24. Preminger GM, Knupp CL, Hindsley JP, Jenkins JM, Fried FA, Blatt PM (1984) Spontaneously acquired anti-factor VIII antibodies: report of a patient with adenocarcinoma of the prostate. J Urol 131:1182–1184
25. Scharrer I (1986) Erworbene Antikörper gegen Gerinnungsfaktoren. Hämostaseologie 6:89–92
26. Schwertfeger R, Hintz G, Huhn D (1991) Successful treatment of a patient with postpartum factor VIII inhibitor with recombinant human Interferon alfa 2a. Am J Hematol 37:190–193
27. Seremetis SV (1994) The Clinical Use of Factor VIIa in the Treatment of Factor VIII Inhibitor Patients. Semin Hematol 31/2 [Suppl 4]:53–55
28. Sultan MD, Kazatchkine MD, Algiman M, Dietrich G, Nydegger U (1993) The Use of Intravenous Immunoglobulins in the Treatment of Factor VIII Inhibitors. Semin Hematol 31/2 [Suppl 4]:65–66
29. Withe GC (1994) Factor VIII Inhibitor Assay: Quantitative and Qualitative Assay Limitations and Development Needs. Semin Hematol 31/2 [Suppl 4]:6

CHAPTER 4

Lupus Anticoagulants

B. Pötzsch

Summary

Lupus anticoagulants are a heterogeneous group of autoantibodies directed against hemostatically active phospholipids and phospholipid-protein complexes. The presence of lupus anticoagulants can predispose to thrombosis and recurrent abortion. Both arterial and venous thrombosis have been described. Reduced anticoagulant activity of activated protein C has been discussed as a possible pathophysiologic mechanism. Various functional and immunologic tests are available for detecting lupus anticoagulants. The definitive diagnosis of a lupus anticoagulant requires a positive result in two independent functional tests or the simultaneous detection of a lupus anticoagulant in one functional and one immunologic test. Treatment aims at the prevention of thromboembolic complications, so patients should remain on oral anticoagulation until lupus anticoagulant parameters have normalized.

Introduction

A lupus anticoagulant (LAC) is an autoantibody directed against hemostatically active phospholipids or phospholipid-protein complexes [5]. In vitro, LAC antibodies lead to a prolongation of phospholipid-dependent coagulation parameters. This phenomenon, which is probably due to competition of LAC antibodies with vitamin-K-dependent coagulation factors for available phospholipid binding sites [8], has led to the term "anticoagulant." In reality, however, circulating LAC antibody does not act as an anticoagulant but is associated with an increased risk of thrombosis and recurrent fetal loss [5].

Clinical Features

Though first described in patients with systemic lupus erythematosus [3, 7], the presence of an LAC does not relate to a particular underlying disease. Indeed, clinical studies prove that no association with an autoimmune disorder or any other systemic disease can be demonstrated in the majority of patients with LACs [6]. Thrombotic events triggered by LACs may involve venous or arterial vessels and may occur at the microcirculatory level. No precise data are available on the relative frequencies of arterial and venous thromboses. It is generally agreed, however, that venous thrombosis is significantly more common than arterial thrombosis. The latter may involve the coronary and cerebral arteries, predisposing to myocardial infarction (MI) and stroke [1]. LAC screening should definitely be performed in young MI patients whose coronary angiograms show no evidence of coronary heart disease [2]. The relatively high incidence of recurrent fetal loss in pregnant women with LACs is attributed to thrombotic occlusion of the placental microcirculation. Another possible symptom of LACs is thrombocytopenia. Normal platelet counts do not exclude the presence of LACs, however, just as thrombocytopenia in an LAC patient is not necessarily caused by the LAC, and a thorough differential diagnosis is always required.

Pathophysiology

The exact mechanism by which LACs predispose to thrombosis is poorly understood. It has been postulated that LAC antibodies bind to the luminal surface of endothelial cells and thereby alter prostacyclin synthesis or the thrombin-thrombomodulin interaction leading to protein C activation, but this has not been confirmed by experimental studies with cultured endothelial cells or by measurements of thromboxane and prostacyclin levels in LAC patients [4, 9]. Moreover, it has been shown that increased concentrations of LAC antibodies do not bind to cultured endothelial cells in comparison with control immunoglobulin. Various groups of authors have demonstrated impaired anticoagulant activity of activated protein C in the presence of LAC antibodies both in cultured endothelium and within the plasma system [4, 9]. It is likely that the LAC antibodies produce this effect by directly competing with the components of the protein C complex for binding sites on the phospholipid surface. Given the limited number of hemostatically active phospholipids that are available in the region of the intact vessel wall, this mechanism could be a major cause of the thrombophilia that exists in patients with LACs [10].

Diagnosis

Both functional and immunologic assay methods can be used in the detection of LACs. In the functional assays, the phospholipids available in the test sample become the limiting quantity, so the prolongation of measured clotting times is directly proportional to the concentration of LAC antibodies in the sample. This principle accounts for the differences in sensitivity among different methods. For example, the more phospholipids are added to an aPTT reagent, the less sensitive the reagent is in detecting an LAC. For this reason, patients with clinical suspicion of an LAC should always undergo two screening tests, such as the LAC-sensitive aPTT combined with the kaolin clotting time (KCT). In the KCT, phospholipid-free kaolin is used as a surface activator. A factor deficiency can be distinguished from the presence of an LAC by the simultaneous analysis of a 1:1 mixture of patient plasma with normal plasma. A disadvantage of this method is its heparin sensitivity, so any heparin present in the plasma sample must be neutralized or enzymatically degraded prior to analysis. Another sensitive screening test that can be used in heparin-containing plasma samples is the textarin/ecarin ratio. While prothrombin activation by textarin is phospholipid-dependent, ecarin activates prothrombin in a cofactor-independent fashion. Thus, LAC antibodies prolong the textarin time but not the ecarin time.

Positive findings in one of the LAC screening tests must be verified by a confirmatory test before a final diagnosis is made. In most confirmatory tests, purified phospholipids or phospholipid-rich fractions are added to the patient's plasma. One test based on this method is the hexagonal (II) phase phospholipid assay described by Rauch et al. in 1989 [11]. In the immunologic assays, phospholipid/β_2 microglobulin mixtures are immobilized on a microtiter plate, covered with the patient's plasma, and bound autoantibodies are assayed using an antibody directed against human immunoglobulins. This method permits a quantitative determination of LAC antibodies. Coating the microtiter plate with the phospholipids poses a technical problem, however, for many hemostatically active phospholipids change their conformation during the coating process and are no longer recognized by LAC antibodies. There are well standardized ELISA tests available for the assay of cardiolipin antibodies. While anticardiolipin antibodies are not identical to LACs, both autoantibodies coexist in many patients, and the determination of anticardiolipin antibodies can be helpful in making a diagnostic and therapeutic assessment.

The quality of the LAC workup depends critically on the preanalytic treatment of the samples. A basic rule is that blood samples should be processed soon after they are drawn. Because platelets provide an "unwanted" source of phospholipids in all functional test procedures, the plasma sample should be centrifuged twice, or centrifuged at 5000 g, to remove the platelets. In heparin-sensitive methods, heparin can be eliminated by preanalytic enzymatic inactivation without compromising the accuracy of the assay. LAC screening should be performed in all patients with unexplained thrombophilia, in patients with a documented autoimmune disease, in women prone to recurrent fetal loss, and in patients with unexplained prolongation of the aPPT.

Treatment

At present there is no causal treatment available for the immunologic defect responsible for the LAC. The goal of treatment, then, is the prevention of thrombotic complications. Patients with confirmed LACs and a positive history of thrombosis should remain on oral anticoagulation until LAC parameters have normalized. The goal is to achieve an INR (international normalized ratio) of 3.0–4.0. The decision for oral anticoagulation is more difficult in patients with confirmed LACs who have had no previous thrombotic events. Although there is still no proof of a definite correlation between the assayed concentration of LAC antibodies and the actual risk of thrombosis, the decision for oral anticoagulation in such cases should depend on the concentration of the LAC antibodies and the presence of additional risk factors. Low-dose heparin therapy should be instituted at once in all patients with documented LACs who are not receiving oral anticoagulation and in patients who are immobilized for a prolonged period or placed in any other situation predisposing to thrombosis. Treatment with platelet aggregation inhibitors is appropriate only in LAC patients with a prior history of arterial thrombosis. Immunosuppressant therapy in LAC patients is indicated only if thrombophilia cannot be controlled with anticoagulant therapy alone. This has been described in a few patients with recurrent pulmonary embolism.

Bleeding in LAC patients is a very rare problem that is treated by administering platelet concentrates. This is indicated even in the absence of thrombocytopenia.

In women with LACs, microthrombosis in the placental circulation can lead to recurrent fetal loss that typically occurs between weeks 12 and 20 of pregnancy. Various case reports and our own experience confirm that the early initiation of anticoagulant therapy will enable many patients to have a successful pregnancy outcome. Ideally the therapy should be initiated before conception. The goal is to achieve plasma levels of 0.3 to 0.4 anti-FXa units. Low-molecular-weight heparins are excellent for this purpose owing to their long half-life. After delivery, nursing mothers should remain on heparin prophylaxis while nonnursing women should be placed on oral anticoagulation for the prevention of thrombosis.

References

1. Baker WF, Bick RL (1994) Antiphospholipid antibodies in coronary artery disease: A review. Semin Thromb Haemost 20:27–45
2. Bick RL, Ishmail Y, Baker WF (1993) Coagulation abnormalities in precocious artery thrombosis and in patients failing coronary artery bypass grafting and percutaneous transcoronary. Semin Thromb Haemost 10:412–417
3. Conley CL, Hartmann R (1952) Hemorrhagic disorder caused by circulating anticoagulant in patients with disseminated lupus erythematosus. J Clin Invest 150:621–622
4. Dudley DJ, Mitchell MD, Branch DW (1990) Pathophysiology of antiphospholipid antibodies: Absence of prostaglandin-mediated effects on cultured endothelium. Am J Obstet Gynecol 162:953–959
5. Feinstein DI (1982) Lupus anticoagulant, anticardiolipin antibodies, fetal loss, and systemic lupus erythematosus. Blood 80:859–862
6. Kornberg A, Silber L, Yona R, Kaufman S (1989) Clinical manifestations and laboratory findings in patients with lupus anticoagulants. Eur J Haematol 42:90–95
7. Mueller JF, Ratnoff O, Heinle RW (1951) Observations on the characteristics of an unusual circulating anticoagulant. Lab Clin Med 38:254–261
8. Pengo V, Thiagarajan P, Shapiro SS, Heine MJ (1987) Immunological specificity and mechanism of action of IgG lupus anticoagulants. Blood 70:69–76
9. Pötzsch B, Kawamura H, Preissner KT et al (1992) Thrombophilia in patients with lupus anticoagulant correlates with impaired anticoagulant activity of activated protein C but not with decreased activation of protein C. Blood 80:267a (Abstract)
10. Pötzsch B, Kawamura H, Preissner KT, Schmidt M, Seelig C, Müller-Berghaus G (1995) Acquired protein C dysfunction but not decreased activity of thrombomodulin is a possible marker of thrombophilia in patients with lupus anticoagulant. J Lab Clin Med 125:56–65
11. Rauch J, Tannenbaum M, Janoff AS (1989) Distinguishing plasma lupus anticoagulants from anti-factor antibodies using hexagonal (II) phase phospholipids. Thromb Haemost 62:892–896

CHAPTER 5

Heparin-Induced Thrombocytopenia

A. Greinacher

Summary

Heparin-induced thrombocytopenia (HIT) is among the most serious potential complications of heparin therapy. Two forms are recognized: a nonimmunologic type I HIT, which causes a slight reduction in platelet counts with no clinical symptoms, and a less common immunologic type II HIT, which may be associated with thromboembolic complications.

In patients without prior exposure to heparin, type II HIT appears from 5 to 20 days after the start of heparin therapy, showing a peak incidence on day 10. If there has been prior heparin exposure, clinical symptoms may appear more rapidly. Type II HIT should be excluded in patients whose platelet counts fall by more than 50% of the initial level after several days' heparin therapy and/or in patients who develop new thromboembolic complications during or shortly after the conclusion of heparin administration. The incidence of type II HIT is 0.5%–2%. The greatest risk to patients is from new vascular occlusions.

The principal antigen of type II HIT is a multimolecular complex composed of platelet factor 4 and heparin. The HIT antibodies bind to platelets and activate them via their Fc component and platelet Fc receptor II. HIT antibodies also bind to and activate endothelial cells. The concurrent activation of platelets and endothelial cells is a likely explanation for the unusual clinical course of type II HIT. Several sensitive laboratory tests are available for confirming the presumptive clinical diagnosis. The low-sulfated heparinoid danaparoid sodium (Orgaran) and recombinant hirudin are the main drugs used for the continued parenteral anticoagulation of affected patients.

Besides hemorrhagic complications, heparin-induced thrombocytopenia (HIT) is the most important adverse effect of heparin therapy. Some authors use the term heparin-associated thrombocytopenia (HAT) or thrombosis-thrombocytopenia syndrome. Despite the nonuniform terminology, authors who work with HIT agree that heparin can induce two forms of thrombocytopenia: a common nonimmunologic form, characterized by slightly reduced platelet counts and no significant clinical symptoms, and an immunologic form, which may be associated with thromboembolic complications [6, 7].

In approximately 10% of patients who receive intravenous heparin (20 000 IU/day), platelet counts fall slightly during the first days of treatment. Rarely, the counts fall below 100 000 platelets/ml and often return to normal despite continued heparin use. This type I HIT is based on direct heparin-platelet interactions.

The capacity of heparins and other sulfated sugars to bind to platelets depends on their molecular weight and degree of sulfatization [24, 33, 34, 38] and on the prior degree of platelet activation [23]. The greater the degree of prior platelet activation, the greater their binding capacity for heparin.

Of all the platelet proteins, platelet factor 4 (PF_4) has the highest affinity for heparin [5, 21]. But heparin also binds to other platelet proteins such as glycoprotein complex IIb/IIIa and Ib/IX.

Platelet activation by heparin depends directly on the molecular weight of the heparin and its degree of sulfatization. It also depends on its AT III binding affinity [4, 36, 39]. The most likely reason for this is an indirect inhibition of adenylate cyclase by heparin after it has bound to the platelets. This reduces the intraplatelet levels of cyclic adenosine monophosphate, with the result that the platelets are more easily activated, and platelet consumption is increased. If the underlying disease itself causes platelet activation, as in unstable angina pectoris, both effects combine to produce a moderate reduction of platelet counts in type I HIT.

Low-molecular-weight heparins (LMWH) and low-sulfated heparinoids bind more weakly to platelets than unfractionated heparin (UFH). It is possible that type I HIT occurs less frequently in patients treated with LMWH than with UFH. We may also assume that nonimmunologic heparin-platelet interactions are important in the pathogenesis of the immunologic type II form of HIT.

Type II HIT, unlike the type I form, occurs from 5 to 20 days after the start of heparin administration. In most patients who have no previous exposure to heparin, complications arise on about day 10. If there has been previous heparin exposure, type II HIT can appear more rapidly after reexposure to heparin [1, 28]. The interval since the first cycle of heparin therapy appears to be an important factor. Patients who have received heparin during the past 12 months are at greatest risk for developing type II HIT when reexposed to heparin.

Most patients respond with a marked fall of platelet counts. The relative decrease in platelets is more important than the absolute platelet count. In the absence of any other underlying disease such as sepsis, type II HIT should be considered in the differential diagnosis of patients whose platelet counts fall by more than 50% during heparin administration. In some patients, however, thromboembolic complications of type II HIT develop before there is a measurable fall in platelet counts. In rare cases platelet counts remain unchanged despite the occurrence of thromboembolic complications.

Thus, the immunologic form of HIT should be excluded in any patient who develops thromboembolic vascular occlusions during or shortly after the completion of heparin administration.

Platelet counts in most patients will return to normal within 7–10 days after the discontinuation of heparin.

Type II HIT is different from all other immune-related thrombocytopenias. Despite parenteral anticoagulation and low platelet counts, bleeding problems are rare. The main risk to patients is the potential for the development of new vascular occlusions in response to heparin administration. Many of these occlusions are caused by white clots composed of platelets, giving rise to the alternate term "white clot syndrome" for type II HIT.

While arterial occlusions have been widely cited in the literature as the hallmark of type II HIT, venous thrombosis and pulmonary embolism were much more common occurrences in the patients diagnosed at our laboratory. Warkentin and Kelton [41] described similar findings. New thromboembolic complications are especially likely to occur in cases where heparin administration is continued after the initial vascular occlusion. These complications have up to a 20% mortality, and there is an equal incidence of incomplete recovery. Limb amputations and neurologic deficits following stroke are the most common sequelae [1, 27, 28, 41].

The immunologic form of HIT is defined by the presence of heparin-dependent antibodies. But since few laboratories employ sensitive diagnostic test procedures such as the ^{14}C serotonin release test [37], the heparin-induced platelet activation test (HIPA [15]), or the PF_4/heparin ELISA assay [2, 18], the true incidence of the antibodies remains unclear.

The most comprehensive data to date on the prevalence of HIT come from a meta-analysis of all prospective studies done prior to 1990 [41]. According to this analysis, high-dose heparin therapy is associated with a greater incidence of HIT than low-dose heparin administration for thromboprophylaxis. The predicted incidence of type II HIT is 0.5%–2% in patients who remain on heparin therapy for more than 5 days. But even the low heparin doses usually administered for thromboprophylaxis can trigger type II HIT [1, 12, 16]. Consistent with the findings in most of the patients diagnosed at our laboratory, Laster et al. report that low-dose heparin administration for thromboprophylaxis induced type II HIT in 82% of their 169 patients [29]. The first prospective study on the incidence of type II HIT using a sensitive laboratory test demonstrated HIT antibodies in 7.4% of all patients who received unfractionated heparin for thromboprophylaxis; 2.8% of these patients showed thrombocytopenia, and 85% developed thrombosis. HIT antibodies were detected in just 2.4% of the patients who received LMWH, and none of the patients showed thrombocytopenia or thrombosis [42]. It is the author's impression that the incidence and the clinical manifestations of type II HIT are dependent on the patient's underlying disease. The incidence of type II HIT appears to be greater than 2% in patients with preexisting vascular disease [20, 35].

Type II HIT also differs from other immune thrombocytopenias in its pathogenic mechanism. Intravascular, heparin-dependent platelet aggregation is a more likely explanation for the thrombocytopenia than the phagocytosis of antibody-laden platelets by the reticuloendothelial system.

The Fc receptor on the platelet surface (FcgRII, CD_{32}) plays a special role in antibody-dependent platelet activation. HIT antibodies bind to platelets via their Fc component; binding to the FcgRII receptor induces platelet activation [3, 9, 17, 26]. HIT antibodies also bind to endothelial cells and activate them [11, 19]. HIT antibodies are not heparin-specific. Amiral et al. [2] were the first to show that HIT antibodies bind to PF_4/heparin complexes. Based on this observation, we were able to characterize multimolecular PF_4/heparin complexes composed of approximately 8 PF_4 molecules per heparin molecule as the principal antigen of type II HIT [11, 19, 40], and we have demonstrated these antigen complexes on platelets and on endothelial cells.

According to the current concept of the pathogenic mechanism of type II HIT, the binding of heparin to platelets depends on its degree of sulfatization and its molecular weight. Heparin activates platelets through multifactorial, nonimmunologic mechanisms.

This proaggregational effect of heparin causes platelet proteins with a heparin binding site to be released from the alpha granules and form multimolecular complexes with heparin and other polysulfated oligosaccharides. The complexes composed of soluble platelet proteins and heparin owe their formation to the strong negative charge of polysulfated oligosaccharides, which also enables them to bind to the platelet surface.

Some patient become immunized to these complexes. In approximately 80% of cases, the immunity is directed against complexes composed of PF_4 and heparin. The multimolecular antigen complexes can probably bind several antibodies, forming immune complexes that activate the platelets via their Fc receptors. Antigen epitopes also form on the surface of endothelial cells. The concurrent activation of platelets and endothelial cells is probably a major factor in the development of thromboembolic complications in patients with type II HIT.

This concept implies a close association between the nonimmunologic type I HIT and the immunologic type II HIT [14]. UFH and high-sulfated heparinoids with a high molecular weight bind more strongly to platelets and are more likely to activate them than LMWH or low-sulfated heparinoids. Owing to their size they can bind more PF_4 tetramers, so they can probably form larger PF_4-heparin complexes.

Accordingly, UFH and high-sulfated heparinoids should have a greater tendency to induce patient immunization and HIT antibody formation than LMWH or low-sulfated heparinoids. This notion is supported by a prospective study in which HIT antibodies were detected less frequently in patients treated with LMWH than with UFH [42].

But in cases where immunization has occurred, LMWHs are as likely as UFHs to form an HIT antigen. This has been shown by several studies that demonstrated almost 100% cross-reactivity of LMWH with HIT antibodies using sensitive in vitro procedures [16, 18]. The degree to which LMWHs induce clinically significant thrombocytopenia or thromboembolic complications in patients with HIT antibodies depends on individual patient characteristics, with comedications (e.g., ASS) and underlying diseases (e.g., preexisting vascular disease) playing an important role.

Because LMWHs can trigger life-threatening complications in patients with type II HIT [13, 22, 30, 31], and because current laboratory tests do not take into account the individual factors noted above, the use of LMWH is absolutely contraindicated in patients with type II HIT.

Consistent with the results of in vitro studies, low-sulfated heparinoids such as danaparoid sodium (Org 10172, Orgaran, AKZO-Organon, The Netherlands) are better suited for the continued parenteral anticoagulation of type II HIT patients. Danaparoid has shown in vitro cross-reactivity in 10%–20% of patients, however [8, 10, 16, 18]. In the largest review to date covering more than 230 type II HIT patients treated with danaparoid, a clinically significant cross-reaction occurred in only 2%–3% of the cases [32]. Recombinant hirudin will provide an important new option in the treatment of patients with type II HIT. Hirudin is an effective platelet inhibitor whose protein structure precludes any cross-reactivity with HIT antibodies. We are presently conducting a multi-center, prospective study to evaluate the efficacy of hirudin in the treatment of patients with type II HIT.

Ancrod, a fibrinogen-degrading snake venom extract, is used in North America for anticoagulation in patients with type II HIT. Because ancrod takes about 24 h to act, does not inhibit thrombin formation, and can cause severe hemorrhagic complications and allergic reactions, very stringent criteria should be followed in selecting patients for this therapy.

The prompt initiation of oral anticoagulants is dangerous in patients with type II HIT. Because the half-life of protein C is shorter than that of the procoagulant factors, vitamin K antagonists cause a transient deficiency of protein C.

Thus, oral anticoagulants should be used in type II HIT only after heparin has been discontinued for at least 5 days, and then should be introduced gradually under cover of a compatible parenteral anticoagulant.

To avoid immunization and the formation of type II HIT antibodies, heparin administration should be limited to a period of 5 days whenever possible. In patients who require more prolonged parenteral heparin anticoagulation, platelet counts should be checked daily before and after the fifth day of heparin use. This protocol is necessary for the early detection of type II HIT. If the 1%–2% incidence of type II HIT during low-dose heparinization for thrombo-prophylaxis is confirmed, the high mortality rate of over 10% is unacceptable given the yearly heparin consumption rate in Germany of more than 60 million doses per day.

Sensitive tests are available for the detection of HIT antibodies, and new methods for the effective treatment of HIT patients have been described in recent years.

Today there is an urgent need for prospective studies on identifying patient groups that are at particularly high risk for developing type II HIT and studies exploring the potential advantage of LMWH in reducing the incidence of type II HIT.

Our increasing knowledge about type II HIT should motivate a careful weighing of the risk and benefits of providing parenteral anticoagulation for more than five days. It would be unacceptable, however, to withhold effective thromboprophylaxis from patients who are at moderate or high risk for developing thrombosis.

References

1. AbuRahma AF, Boland JP, Witsberger T (1991) Diagnostic and therapeutic strategies of white clot syndrome. Am J Surg 162:175–179
2. Amiral J, Bridey F, Dreyfus M, Vissac AM, Fressinaud E, Wolf M, Meyer D (1992) Platelet factor 4 complexed to heparin is the target for antibodies generated in heparin-induced thrombocytopenia. Thromb Haemost 68:95–96
3. Anderson GP: Insights into heparin-induced thrombocytopenia. Br J Haematol 80:504–508
4. Brace LD, Fareed J (1985) An objective assessment of the interaction of heparin and its fractions with human platelets. Semin Thromb Hemost 11:190–198
5. Capitanio AM, Niewiarowski S, Rucinski B, Tuszynski GP, Cierniewski CS, Hershock D, Kornecki E (1985) Interaction of platelet factor 4 with human platelets. Biochim Biophys Acta 839:161–173
6. Carreras LO (1980) Thrombosis and thrombocytopenia induced by heparin. Scand J Haematol 25 [Suppl 36]:66–80
7. Chong BH, Berndt MC (1989) Heparin-induced thrombocytopenia. Blut 58:53–57
8. Chong BH, Magnani HN (1992) Orgaran in heparin-induced thrombocytopenia. Haemostasis 22:85–91
9. Chong BH, Fawaz I, Chesterman CN, Berndt MC (1989) Heparin-induced thrombocytopenia: mechanism of interaction of the heparin-dependent antibody with platelets. Br J Haematol 73:235–240
10. Chong BH, Ismail F, Cade J, Gallus AS, Gordon S, Chesterman CN (1989) Heparin-induced thrombocytopenia: studies with a new low molecular weight heparinoid, Org 10172. Blood 73:1592–1596
11. Cines DB, Tomaski A, Tannenbaum S (1987) Immune endothelial-cell injury in heparin-associated thrombocytopenia. N Engl J Med 316:581–589
12. Demers C, Ginsberg JS, Brill-Edwards P, Panju A, Warkentin TE, Anderson DR, Turner C, Kelton JG (1991) Rapid anticoagulation using ancrod for heparin-induced thrombocytopenia. Blood 78:2194–2197
13. Eichinger S, Kyrle P, Breuner B, Wagner B, Kapiotis S, Lechner K, Korininger HC (1991) Thrombocytopenia associated with low-molecular-weight heparin. Lancet 337:1425–1426
14. Greinacher A (1995) The nonimmunologic type I and the immunologic type II of heparin associated thrombocytopenia are closely linked in their pathogenesis. Sem Thromb Hemost 21:106–116
15. Greinacher A, Michels I, Kiefel V, Mueller-Eckhardt C (1991) A rapid and sensitive test for diagnosing heparin-associated thrombocytopenia. Thromb Haemost 66:734–736
16. Greinacher A, Michels I, Mueller-Eckhardt C (1992) Heparin-associated thrombocytopenia: the antibody is not heparin specific. Thromb Haemost 67:545–549
17. Greinacher A, Michels I, Liebenhoff U, Presek P, Mueller-Eckhardt C (1993) Heparin-associated thrombocytopenia: immune complexes are attached to the platelet membrane by the negative charge of highly sulfated oligosaccharides. Br J Haematol 84:711–716
18. Greinacher A, Amiral J, Dummel V, Vissac AM, Kiefel V, Mueller-Eckhardt C (1994) Laboratory diagnosis of heparin-associated thrombocytopenia, comparison of platelet aggregation test, heparin-induced platelet activation (HIPA) test, and PF4/heparin ELISA. Transfusion 34:381–385
19. Greinacher A, Pötzsch B, Amiral J, Dummel V, Eichner A, Mueller-Eckhardt C (1994) Heparin-associated thrombocytopenia: isolation of the antibody and characterization of a multimolecular PF4-heparin complex as the major antigen. Thromb Haemost 71:247–251
20. Hach-Wunderle V, Kainer K, Salzmann G, Müller-Berghaus G, Pötzsch B (1995) Heparin-associated thrombosis despite normal platelet counts. Ann Hematol 70 [Suppl 1]: A 56
21. Handin RI, Cohen HJ (1976) Purification and binding properties of human platelet factor four. J Biol Chem 251:4273–4282
22. Horellou MH, Conard J, Lecrubier C, Samama M, Roque D, Orbcastel O, Fenoyl O de, diMaria G, Bernadou A (1984) Persistent heparin induced thrombocytopenia despite therapy with low molecular weight heparin. Thromb Haemost 51:134

23. Horne MK, Chao ES (1989) Heparin binding to rested and activited platelets. Blood 74:238–243
24. Horne MK, Chao ES (1990) The effect of molecular weight on heparin binding to platelets. Br J Haematol 74:306–312
25. Kelton JG (1986) Heparin-induced thrombocytopenia. Haemostasis 16:173–186
26. Kelton JG, Sheridan D, Santos A, Smith J, Steeves K, Smith C, Brown C, Murphy WG (1988) Heparin-induced thrombocytopenia: laboratory studies. Blood 72:925–930
27. King DJ, Kelton JG (1984) Heparin-associated thrombocytopenia. Ann Intern Med 100:535–540
28. Kleinschmidt S, Ziegenfuß T, Seyfert UT, Greinacher A (1993) Septisch-toxisches Herz-Kreislauf-Versagen als Folge einer Heparin-induzierten Thrombozytopenie mit „White-Clot-Syndrome". Anästh Intensivther Notfallmed 28:58–60
29. Laster J, Cikrit D, Walker N, Silver D (1987) The heparin-induced thrombocytopenia syndrome: an update. Surgery 102:763–770
30. Lecompte T, Luo SK, Stieltjes N, Lecrubier C, Samama MM (1991) Thrombocytopenia associated with low-molecular-weight heparin. Lancet 338:1217
31. Leroy J, Leclerc MH, Delahousse B, Guerois C, Foloppe P, Gruel Y, Toulemonde F (1985) Treatment of heparin-associated thrombocytopenia and thrombosis with low molecular weight heparin (CY 216). Semin Thromb Hemost 11:326–329
32. Magnani HN (1993) Heparin-induced thrombocytopenia: an overview of 230 patients treated with orgaran (Org 10172). Thromb Haemost 70:554–561
33. Messmore HL, Griffin B, Fareed J, Coyne E, Seghatchian J (1989) In vitro studies of the interaction of heparin, low molecular weight heparin and heparinoids with platelets. Ann NY Acad Sci 556:217–232
34. Messmore HL, Griffin B, Koza M, Seghatchian J, Fareed J, Coyne E (1989) Interaction of heparinoids with platelets: comparison with heparin and low molecular weight heparins. Semin Thromb Hemost 17 [Suppl] 1:57–59
35. Reininger CB, Reininger AJ, Steckmeier B, Laser R, Schweiberer A, Greinacher A (1995) Platelet hypersensitivity to heparin and increased incidence of heparin-induced thrombocytopenia (HIT) in leg atherosclerosis. Ann hematol 70 [Suppl 1]: A51
36. Salzman EW, Rosenberg RD, Smith MH, Lindon JN, Favreau L (1980) Effect of heparin and heparin fractions on platelet aggregation. J Clin Invest 65:64–73
37. Sheridan D, Carter C, Kelton JG (1986) A diagnostic test for heparin-induced thrombocytopenia. Blood 67:27–30
38. Sobel M, Adelman B (1988) Characterization of platelet binding of heparins and other glycosaminoglycans. Thromb Res 50:815–826
39. Vermylen JG (1993) Effect of heparin and low molecular weight heparins on platelets. Semin Thromb Hemost 19 [Suppl 1]:20–21
40. Visentin GP, Ford SE, Scott JP, Aster RH (1994) Antibodies from patients with heparin-induced thrombocytopenia/thrombosis are specific for platelet factor 4 complexe with heparin or bound to endothelial cells. J Clin Invest 93:81–88
41. Warkentin TE, Kelton JG (1991) Heparin-induced thrombocytopenia. Prog Hemost Thromb 10:1–34
42. Warkentin TE, Levine MN, Roberts RS, Gent M, Horsewood P, Kelton JG (1993) Heparin-induced thrombocytopenia is more common with unfractionated heparin than with low molecular weight heparin. Thromb Haemost 69:911

Part III

Massive Bleeding

CHAPTER 6

Bleeding in Transplantation Surgery

H. RIESS

Summary

Bleeding complications in transplantation surgery result both from the complexity of the operation and from specific hemostatic changes caused by the underlying organ defect. Thus, in the absence of secondary organ damage, the risk of bleeding in cardiac transplantation is basically the same as in coronary bypass surgery. The hemostatic defect that occurs as a result of decompensated heart failure with consequent multiple organ failure, sometimes aggravated by extracorporeal cardiopulmonary bypass with anticoagulation, greatly compounds the risk of bleeding during the subsequent transplantation. While we are just beginning to understand the pathophysiology of these problems and their therapeutic implications, we have a much better awareness of the problems involved in liver transplantation. We shall also consider bone marrow transplantation, whose basic principles differ substantially from those of solid organ transplantations.

Liver Transplantation

The liver plays a central role in the hemostasis system, functioning as the primary site for the synthesis of coagulation and fibrinolytic factors and important protease inhibitors. In addition, the reticuloendothelial system of the liver contributes to the clearance of activated hemostasis factors and their complexes with inhibitors.

Liver transplantation (usually orthotopic) causes further hemostatic changes in a patient who already has hemostatic abnormalities as a result of liver disease. These changes are manifested chiefly by diffuse intra- and post-operative bleeding with blood loss greater than would be expected from portal hypertension, and they occur almost exclusively in the reperfusion phase of the liver transplantation [3, 8, 12, 24].

Mediators released into the circulation from the surgical wounds and host liver (preanhepatic and anhepatic phases) and from the perfused donor liver presumably contribute as much to worsening the preexisting hemostatic defects as the contact of the blood with foreign surfaces in the extracorporeal portosystemic bypass system and the perioperative administration of drugs and blood products.

Plasmatic Hemostasis and Liver Transplantation

While earlier studies in the anhepatic phase of liver transplantation showed marked signs of increased activation of the coagulation system with a decrease in clotting factors, inhibitors, and platelets [3, 8], more recent studies [9, 12, 24] using improved anesthetic and surgical techniques and a lower transfusion requirement have shown little or no evidence of this. Various groups of authors have consistently found that reperfusion of the liver graft is associated with a marked activation of coagulation leading to elevated levels of thrombin-antithrombin III complexes and fibrin monomers accompanied by reduced levels of fibrinogen, antithrombin III, protein C, and C1 inhibitor. These findings document an increased activation of prothrombin and fibrinogen after graft reperfusion, following the pattern of an incipient, disseminated intravascular consumption coagulopathy. With an uncomplicated transplantation, a significant rise in protein C activity and fibrinogen can be measured within 12 h after reperfusion as an expression of the synthetic function of the liver [12].

As early as the 1960s, studies based on thromboelastography (TEG) and euglobulin clot lysis time suggested the importance of increased fibrinolytic activity during liver transplantations. More recent studies [6, 12, 13, 24] show that the activity of tissue plasminogen activator (tPA) increases markedly during the anhepatic phase and is maximal at the start of the reperfusion phase. This rise in tPA activity is paralleled by an increase in the activity of intrinsic plasminogen activators. This accounts for the TEG signs of hyperfibrinolysis and the observed increases in plasmin-α_2-antiplasmin complexes and, to a lesser degree, D dimers. A rapid decline of tPA and uPA activity occurs in the postanhepatic reperfusion phase. An opposite pattern is seen with plasminogen activator inhibitor (PAI-1), which remains at its initial level during the preanhepatic and anhepatic phases and rises sharply with reperfusion. Clinical studies establish a correlation between an increase in fibrinolysis and the perioperative transfusion requirement.

In summary, the anhepatic phase of orthotopic liver transplantation is marked by increasing fibrinolytic activity (Fig. 1) that gives way to an increasing activation of plasmatic coagulation on graft reperfusion (Fig. 2). The increased activity of the extrinsic and intrinsic fibrinolytic system in the anhepatic period is presumably caused by diminished hepatic clearance of plasminogen activators and the absence of an increase in their inhibitors. While intrinsic activators such as prourokinase are administered with fresh frozen plasma (FFP) during the anhepatic phase in response to the increased volume requirement, the increase in tPA activity is probably a result of increased endothelial release in the operative area. There is no compelling evidence for a secondary mechanism of hyperfibrinolysis, i.e., a previous systemic activation of plasmatic coagulation. The fall in plasma fibrinolytic activity that occurs with reperfusion of the transplanted liver is evidently due to the rapid rise in PAI following graft reperfusion. This may be caused by a release of PAI from activated platelets or from the liver graft during reperfusion.

The importance of leukocytes in the hemostatic disorders of liver transplantation is evidenced by the demonstration of lysosomal proteases released from granulocytes (elastase) and macrophages (cathepsin B) and rising levels of tumor necrosis factor and neopterin (Fig. 2 [26, 27]). The elastase-proteinase inhibitor complex rises slightly during the anhepatic phase but shows a marked rise after graft perfusion and remains high for a period of hours after reperfusion. In addition to the elastase released from polymorphocellular granulocytes, there is an extremely sharp postperfusion rise in cathepsin B, which then falls gradually after graft reperfusion. These results strongly suggest that these proteinases or other simultaneously released lysosomal mediators play a key role in the disturbance of hemostasis following revascularization.

Platelets and Liver Transplantation

The fall in the platelet count during the reperfusion phase presumably results from the sequestration of recipient platelets in the transplanted liver. Other factors in platelet reduction after orthotopic liver transplantation may involve platelet consumption in the cold-ischemia-altered vascular system of the donor liver or platelet loss due to postreperfusion activation of the plasmatic coagulation cascade (consumption coagulopathy).

Ex vivo studies of platelet function in platelet-rich plasma with constant platelet numbers have shown a reduction of platelet stimulability that starts immediately after graft reperfusion and persists for more than 60 min [14].

Treatment Options

Insights into the pathogenesis of hemostatic disorders in liver transplantation enhance our understanding of how increased cold ischemic time of the donor liver and in situ "flushing" of the graft correlate with an increased bleeding tendency in transplant recipients.

There is considerable doubt as to whether individualized replacement therapy with FFP and packed RBCs should be routinely supplemented by platelet transfusions or the administration of other concentrates (antithrombin III, PPSB, fibrinogen), and some centers that have an excellent record with liver transplantations categorically reject this approach.

In several studies, synthetic antifibrinolytic agents [4, 17] and aprotinin [13, 19, 21] were found to have a positive effect on the laboratory parameters of increased fibrinolysis (Fig. 3) without increasing the incidence of thromboembolic complications in liver transplantations generally performed without the use of intraoperative heparin [25]. A growing number of studies on the proteinase inhibitor aprotinin are showing that the use of this drug can significantly reduce the intraoperative transfusion requirement (Table 1). Other benefits are a demonstrable reduction in tPA activity and decreased signs of fibrinolysis in the thrombelastogram, depending on the plasma level of aprotinin (Fig. 4). These benefits have prompted the regular use of aprotinin

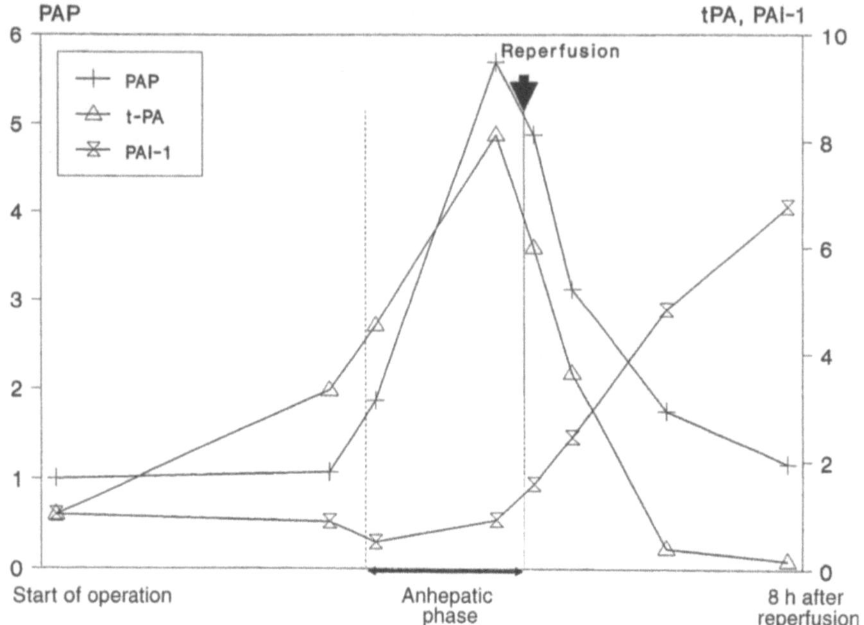

Fig. 1. Relative changes in selected fibrolytic parameters compared with initial values at the start of surgery during the course of orthotopic liver transplantations in 13 adults. *PAI* Plasminogen activator inhibitor activity, *PAP* plasmin-antiplasmin complex, *t-PA* tissue plasminogen activator activity

medication in various liver transplantation centers. Antifibrinolytic agents are frequently effective in patients with overt diffuse bleeding.

Initial studies appear to show that low-dose prostaglandin E1 infusion during liver transplantation can protect against the postreperfusion fall in platelet counts and depression of platelet function without causing an increased bleeding diathesis [11].

The relative importance of the above treatment options in the perioperative management of liver transplantation patients requires further clarification by clinical studies in large numbers of cases.

Bone Marrow Transplantation

Hemostasis problems are common in patients undergoing bone marrow transplantation (BMT). The most frequent problems consist of relatively mild cutaneous and mucosal hemorrhages. Hemorrhagic cystitis is most likely to occur in patients who have been conditioned with busulfan or cyclophosphamide. Severe hemostatic disturbances such as gastrointestinal bleeding, which usually occurs in the setting of graft-versus-host disease (GVHD) of the

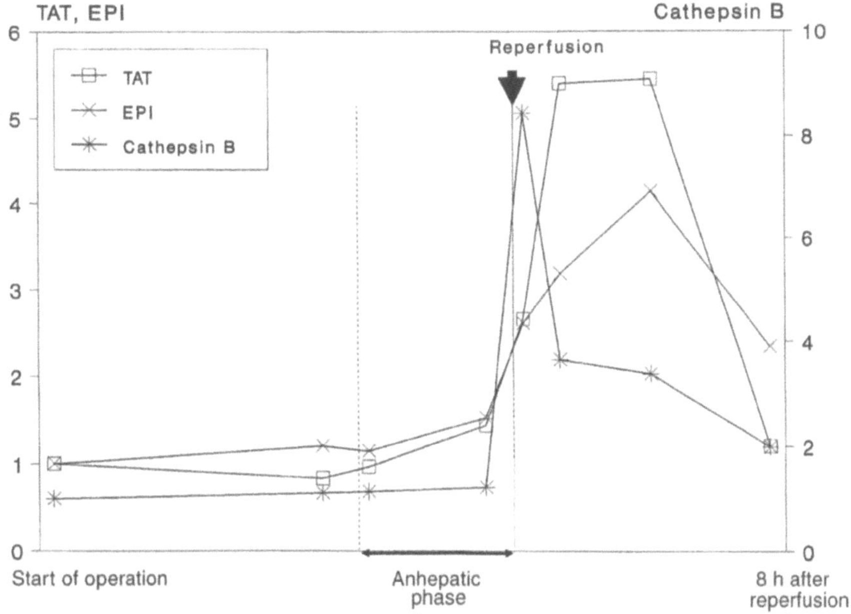

Fig. 2. Relative changes in selected hemostasis parameters compared with initial values at the start of surgery during the course of orthotopic liver transplantations in 13 adults. *EPI* Elastase-proteinase inhibitor complex, *TAT* thrombin-antithrombin III complex, *Cathepsin B* cathepsin B activity (×2)

bowel, central nervous system bleeding, and hemorrhagic myocarditis are rare complications but can be life-threatening or fatal.

Another complication of BMT with a high mortality involving the hemostasis system is veno-occlusive disease (VOD) of the liver.

Platelets and BMT

Thrombocytopenia is considered the major factor underlying hemorrhagic complications. Platelet depression is a consistent postoperative finding that may be transient (initial thrombocytopenia) or may persist following BMT.

Initial Thrombocytopenia

Conditioning with myeloablative chemotherapy or radiation leads to bone marrow aplasia. A rise in leukocytes should occur within about 15 days after BMT. The resumption of thrombocytopoiesis normally occurs later, at approximately 4 weeks. The period of thrombocytopenia can be bridged by the administration of leukocyte-depleted platelet concentrates, preferably obtained from individual donors. Replacement is indicated in the presence of overt

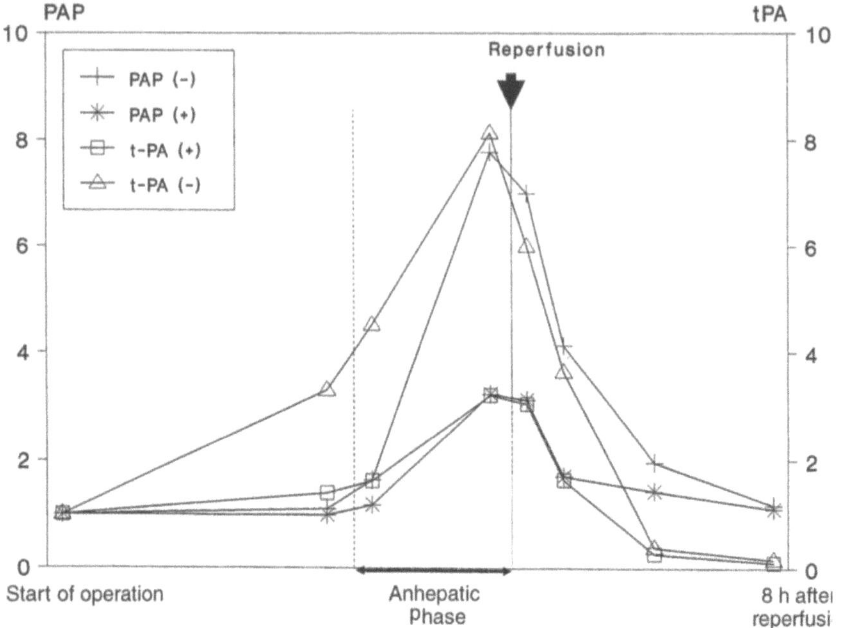

Fig. 3. Relative changes in tissue plasminogen activator activity and the plasmin-antiplasmin complex compared with initial values at the start of surgery during the course of orthotopic liver transplantations with (+) and without (-) aprotonin (200 000 KIU/h) in 10 adult patients

bleeding or when values fall below an empirical cutoff, often defined as a platelet count lower than 10–20 g/l. Special problems exist in patients who, due to antibody formation, react to the platelet concentrates with little or no elevation in platelet counts. Various factors can contribute to a prolongation of the thrombocytopenic phase: Unless the transplantation is successful (engraftment), hematologic recovery will not occur. The success rate of engraftment is better than 99%, however. Infection poses a particular threat during the leukocytopenic phase, and there is a risk of developing a consumption coagulopathy that could intensify or prolong thrombocytopenia. A drug-induced platelet reduction (e.g., by antibiotics or cyclosporin A) should also be considered in the differential diagnosis. Moreover, there have been numerous descriptions of thrombotic-thrombocytopenic purpura (TTP) and hemolytic uremic syndrome (HUS) occurring in the wake of BMT. Conditioning toxicity, GVHD, opportunistic infections, and cyclosporin A immunosuppression have been discussed as pathogenic factors. The prognosis in BMT patients with HUS is poor, with a mortality of 80% [16, 29].

In addition to thrombocytopenia, high-dose chemotherapy is associated with a thrombocytopathy [22] that may result from the drug regimen itself, secondary organic complications, or GVHD.

Table 1. Aprotonin dosage and transfusion requirement in liver transplantations

Authors	Dosage (millions of KIU)	RBC	Control group	RBC	$n(p)$
Bechtstein et al. [2a]	3×0.5	7.5	Historical	9.7	10/10 (s.)
Grosse et al. [7b]	2.0–0.5/h	8.1	Historical	23.3	40/50 (h.s.)
Mallet et al. [19a]	2.0–0.5/h + 0.07/RBC	7.5	Historical	23.6	20/25 (h.s.)
Groh et al. [7a]	2.9–0.5/h	18	Double blind prospective, randomized controlled	20	10/10 (n.s.)
Himmelreich et al. [13]	0.2/h–0.4/h	7	Prospective randomized, 3×0.5	8	10/13 (n.s.)
Ickx et al. [15a]	3.0/h	7	1.5/h (TEG)	7.4	5/5 (n.s.)
Suarez et al. [28a]	2.0–5.0/h	7	Nonrandomized controlled	11.6	13/15 (h.s.)

RBC, units of packed red blood cells.

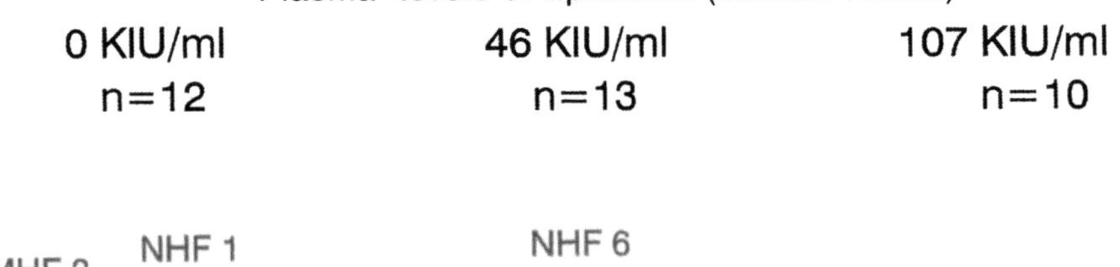

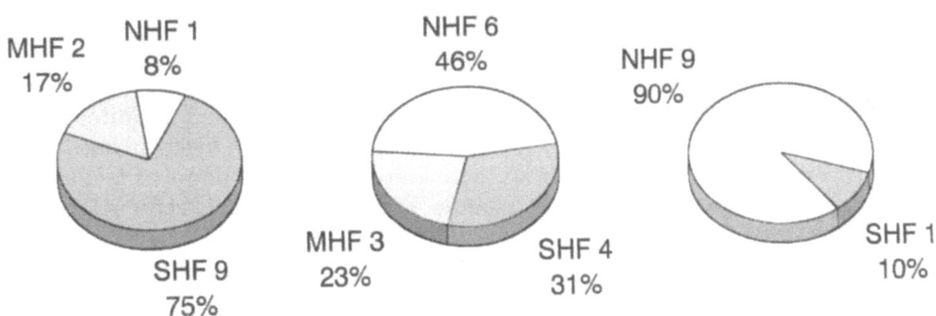

Fig. 4. Degree of increased fibrinolysis in the thrombelastogram at the end of the anhepatic phase, correlated with various plasma levels of aprotonin (expressin in kallikrein inhibitory units, *KIU*). *SHF* Severe hyperfibrinolysis (WBCLT < 90 min), *MHF* mild hyperfibrinolysis (90 min <WBCLT < 120 min), *NHF* no hyperfibrinolysis (WBCLT >120 min); *WBCLT* whole blood clot lysis time

Persistent Thrombocytopenia

Immune and autoimmune processes are of major importance in the persistence of thrombocytopenia after BMT. The development of antibodies that induce thrombocytopenia has been attributed to residual recipient lymphocytes, donor lymphocytes, drugs, altered antigen expression of the bone marrow (e.g., by in vitro treatment), and transfusions. Immune thrombocytopenia may occur up to one year or more after BMT [20, 23]. Also, an immune-mediated functional defect of the progenitor cells may exist in patients with chronic GVHD [1]. The persistent form of thrombocytopenia, which often is associated with GVHD, is considered a poor prognostic sign [7].

Endothelium and BMT

Endothelial cell damage appears to be the central pathogenic mechanism in major complications of BMT such as GVHD, VOD, TTP, and HUS. Tumor necrosis factor α (TNFα) may play an important role as a mediator [15] leading to decreased thrombomodulin expression of the endothelial cell.

Given the presumed relevance of endothelial cell damage, there is an unfortunate lack of methods for the early detection of endothelial abnormalities. So far no laboratory markers have been established clinically for identifying an endothelial cell defect.

Plasmatic Coagulation and BMT

Little research has been done on changes in plasmatic coagulation and the fibrinolytic system following BMT. Treatment and prophylaxis during the aplastic phase, where there is risk of consumption coagulopathy (see above), follow established guidelines. It has been shown that cyclosporin A can trigger the activation of plasmatic coagulation pathways, possibly leading to life-threatening consumption coagulopathy with hyperfibrinolysis [28].

A reduction of factors VII, X, and XII and of protein C and S inhibitors has been described after BMT [5, 10, 18]. The following etiologic mechanisms have been proposed: decreased synthesis, activation, or consumption of factors; a cytostatic-induced disturbance of vitamin K absorption; and factor XII activation by circulating endotoxins.

It is unclear whether the above changes play a role in the development of abnormal bleeding or VOD. The possible benefits of heparin administration in the prevention or treatment of VOD are controversial. The successful use of tPA in the treatment of VOD has been reported [2].

Concluding Remarks

The prevention and treatment of bleeding complications in transplantation surgery have been significantly advanced by an enhanced awareness of underlying pathophysiologic processes. The examples of liver transplantation and bone marrow transplantation show that optimized perioperative approaches to interdisciplinary management with improved techniques for the diagnosis of hemostatic disorders and the selective use of prophylactic hemoreplacement and drug treatment regimens have helped to make transplantation an effective option in the management of critically ill patients.

References

1. Atkinson K, Norrie S, Chan P, Zehnwirth B, Downs K, Biggs J (1986) Hematopoietic progenitor cell function after HLA-identical sibbling bone marrow transplantation: Influence of chronic graft-versus-host disease. Int J Cell Cloning 4:203
2. Baglin TP, Harper P, Marcus RE (1990) Venoocclusive disease of the liver complicating ABMT successfully treated with recombinant tissue plasminogen activator (rt-PA). Bone Marrow Transplan 5:439–441
2a. Bechstein WO, Riess H, Neuhaus P, Himmelreich G, Steffen R, Slama KJ, Rossaint R, Blumhardt G (1991) The effect of aprotinin on blood product requirements during orthotopic liver transplantation. Clin Transplant 5:422–426
3. Böhming HJ (1977) The coagulation disorder of orthotopic hepatic transplantation. Semin Thromb Hemostasis 4:57–82
4. Col-De Beys C, Carlier M, Reynaert M, Lavenne-Pardonge E, Legrand-Monsieur A, Otte J-B, Moriau M (1991) Prediction of bleeding during orthotopic liver transplantation in recipients given tranexamic acid. Thromb Haemostas 65:1088 [Abstract]
5. Devergie A, Scrobohaci ML, Drouet L, Vilmer E, Gluckman E (1986) Changes in endothelial and coagulation parameters after allogeneic bone marrow transplant (BMT) as a mean of prediction of veinoocclusive disease (VOD). Exp Haematol 14:430 [Abstract]
6. Dzik WH, Arkin CF, Jenkins RL, Stump DC (1988) Fibrinolysis during liver transplantation in humans. Role of tissue-type plasminogen activator. Blood 71:1090–1095
7. First LR, Smith BR, Lipton J, Nathan DG, Parkman R, Rappeport JM (1985) Isolated thrombocytopenia after allogenic bone marrow transplantation: Existence of transient and chronic thrombocytopenic syndromes. Blood 665:368–374
7a. Groh J, Welte M, Azad SC, Forst H, Pratschke E, Kratzer MAA (1992) Does aprotinin affect blood loss in liver transplantation? Lancet 340:173
7b. Grosse H, Lobbes W, Frambach M, von Broen O, Ringe B, Barthels M (1991) The use of high dose aprotinin in liver transplantations. The influence on fibrinolysis and blood loss. Tromb Res 63:287–297
8. Groth CG, Pechet L, Starzl TE (1969) Coagulation during and after orthotopic transplantation of the human liver. Arch Surg 98:31–34
9. Harper PL, Luddington RJ, Jennings L, Reardon D, Seaman MJ, Carrell RW, Klinik JR, Smith M, Rolles K, Calne R (1989) Coagulation changes following hepatic revascularisation during liver transplantation. Transplantation 48:603–607
10. Harper PL, Jarvis J, Jenning I, Luddington R, Marcus RE (1990) Changes in the natural anticoagulants following bone marrow transplantation. Bone Marrow Transplan 5:39–42
11. Himmelreich G, Riess H (1991) In vitro inhibition of platelet aggregation by the liver preservation fluid UW solution. Transplantation 52:30–33
12. Himmelreich G, Kierzek B, Neuhaus P, Slama K-J, Riess H(1991) Coagulation changes and the influence of the early perfusate in the course of orthotopic liver transplantation (OLT) when aprotinin is used introperatively. Blood Coagul Fibrinol 2:51–59
13. Himmelreich G, Muser M, Steffen R, Bechstein WO, Slama K-J, Jochum M, Riess H (im Druck) Different aprotinin applications influencing hemostatic changes in orthotopic liver transplantation (OLT). Transplantation
14. Himmelreich G, Hundt K, Neuhaus P, Roissant R, Riess H (im Druck) Prostaglandine E1 infusion intraoperatively is reducing impaired platelet aggregation after reperfusion in orthotopic liver transplantation. Transplantation
15. Holler E, Kolb HJ, Müller A, Kempeni S, Liesenfeld S, Pechumer H, Lehmacher W, Ruckdeschel W, Gleixner B, Riedner C, Ledderose G, Brehm G, Mittermller J, Wilmanns W (1990) Increased serum levels of tumor necrosis factor o precede major complications of bone marrow transplantation. Blood 75:1011–1016

15a. Ickx et al (1993) Effect of two different dosages of aprotonin on perioperative blood loss during liver transplantation. Semin Thromb Hemostasis Volume 19, No. 3, pp 300–301

16. Juckett M, Perry EH, Daniels BS, Weisdorf DJ (1991) Hemolytic uremic syndrome following bone marrow transplantation. Bone Marrow Transplant 7:405–409

17. Kang YG, Lewis JH, Navalgund A, Russell MW, Bontempo FA, Niren LS, Starzl TE (1987) Epsilon-aminocaproic acid for treatment of fibrinolysis during liver transplantation. Anesthesiology 66:766–773

18. Kaufmann PA, Jones RB, Greenberg CS, Peters WP (1990) Autologous bone marrow transplantation and factor XII, factor VII, and protein C deficiencies. Cancer 66:515–521

19. Le Querrec A, Derlon A, Deshayes JP, Tartiere J, Segol P, Bricard H, Thomas M (1991) Effect of aprotinin on fibrinolysis during orthotopic liver transplantation: a preliminary study. Thromb Haemostas 65:1089 [Abstract]

19a. Mallet SV, Cox D, Burroughs AK, Rolles K (1991) The intra-operative use of Trasylol (aprotinin) in liver transplantation. Transplant Int 4:227–230

20. Minchinton RM, Waters AH (1985) Autoimmune thrombocytopenia and neutropenia after marrow transplantation. Blood 66:752 [Letter]

21. Neuhaus P, Bechstein WO, Lefebre B, Blumhardt G, Slama K (1988) Effect of aprotinin on intraoperative bleeding and fibrinolysis in liver transplantation. Lancet II:1924.14

22. Panella TJ, Peters W, White JG, Hannun YA, Greenberg CS (1990) Platelets acquire a secretion defect after high-dose chemotherapy. Cancer 65:1711–1716

23. Panzer S, Kiefel V, Bartram CR, Haas OA, Hinterberger W, Mueller-Eckardt C, Lechner K (1989) Immune thrombocytopenia more than a year after allogeneic bone marrow transplantation due to antibodies against donor platelets with anti-PlA1 specificity: evidence for a host-derived immune reaction. Br J Hematol 71:259–264

24. Porte RJ, Knot EAR, Bontempo FA (1989) Hemostasis in liver transplantation: a review. Gastroenterology 97:488–501

25. Riess H (1995) The use of aprotinin in liver transplantation. In: Pifarre R (ed) Blood conservation with aprotinin. Hanley & Belfus, Philadelphia, pp 349–358

26. Riess H, Jochum M, Machleidt W, Himmelreich G, Roissaint R, Steffen R (1991) Possible role of extracellularly released phagocyte proteinases in the coagulation disorder during liver transplantation. Transplantation 52:482–490

27. Riess H, Jochum M, Machleidt W, Himmelreich G, Muser M, Huhn D (1991) Tumor necrosis factor: possible role in the disorder of hemostasis during liver transplantation. Thromb Haemostas 65:1091 [Abstract]

28. Smith RE, Berg DD (1988) Coagulation defects in cyclosporine A treated allogeneic bone marrow transplant patients. Am J Hematol 28:137–140

28a. Suarez et al (1993) Effectiveness of aprotonin in orthotopic liver transplantation. Semin Thromb Hemostasis Volume 19, No. 3, 292–296

29. Tschuchnigg M, Bradstock KF, Koutts J, Stewart J, Enno A, Seldon M (1990) A case of thrombotic thrombocytopenic purpura following bone marrow transplantation. Bone Marrow Transplant 5:61–63

CHAPTER 7

Bleeding After Massive Transfusion

M. Köhler

Summary

Surgically intractable diffuse microvascular bleeding (MVB) occurs in approximately 20% of patients who have undergone massive blood transfusion. Standard transfusion regimens up to one blood volume, or approximately 10 U of red cell concentrates (RBCs), probably cannot prevent this complication. There is no evidence to support prophylactic replacement with RBCs or fresh frozen plasma (FFP) up to this degree of blood loss. This is due mainly to the complexity of the hemostatic disturbance. In cases of greater blood loss (multiple blood volumes, or approximately 20 U of RBCs), packed red cells and FFP can be transfused in a 1:1 ratio to limit the extent of the dilutional coagulopathy. Clinical examination raises initial suspicion of this complication. The most frequent cause of MVB is thrombocytopenia or platelet dysfunction. Platelet concentrates should be administered, therefore, when platelet counts fall below 50 000/μl following massive transfusion and hemorrhage. Since these patients also tend to have impaired platelet function, it is occasionally necessary to institute platelet replacement in patients who have higher platelet counts. With a concomitant disturbance of plasmatic hemostasis, the product of first choice is FFP. If the hemostatic impairment is so severe that effective replacement therapy with FFP does not appear feasible (hypervolemia), additional factor concentrates should be administered, most notably PPSB and fibrinogen concentrate (fibrinogen < 0.8 g/l). Since the antithrombin III level is generally depressed as well, and since many patients have DIC, antithrombin III concentrate should be given to correct the deficiency before PPSB is administered. It should also be determined whether low-dose heparin therapy should be provided, and if so, it should be instituted prior to replacement with PPSB or fibrinogen concentrate.

Introduction and Definition

"Massive transfusion" (MT) generally refers to a symptom complex that arises when blood loss equivalent to at least one patient blood volume is treated by the transfusion of stored whole blood or red cell concentrates (10–12 U) within 24 h. The clinical causes that can prompt massive transfusion are diverse. Multiple trauma, ruptured aneurysm, vascular surgery, obstetric hemorrhage, liver transplantation, as well as gastrointestinal hemorrhage are often associated with substantial blood loss. The current survival rate of massively transfused adults is approximately 60% [13].

In addition to the familiar side effects of blood transfusion, MT may be followed by a specific, complex hemostatic disturbance, the principal features of which are a dilutional coagulopathy, thrombocytopenia, platelet dysfunction, disseminated intravascular coagulation (DIC), and microembolism. This disturbance can lead postoperatively to a nonsurgical bleeding diathesis known as diffuse microvascular bleeding (MVB). The reported incidence of MVB is approximately 20%–30%.

In many earlier studies, whole blood or modified whole blood was used for the treatment of massive bleeding. Thus, the results of many studies, mostly from the U.S., are not fully applicable to current circumstances. Whole blood is less stable on storage than modern blood component products such packed RBCs, platelet concentrates (PC), and fresh frozen plasma (FFP). The platelets and leukocytes in stored whole blood rapidly form aggregates that, in the MT setting, can lead to microembolism and consequent impairment of pulmonary function (ARDS). Some hemostasis factors (factor V, factor VIII, von Willebrand factor) are also unstable in stored whole blood, falling to about 25% of their initial levels within a few hours.

Leukocytes in RBCs are reduced by 90%, while platelets and even the labile hemostasis factors have normal activities in their respective products (PC and FFP). Given the transfusion schemes currently used in Germany, however, it should be noted that the exclusive use of RBCs in additive solution containing only minute amounts of plasma is associated with a greater dilution of hemostasis factors than the use of whole blood.

Below we shall review the factors leading to the complex coagulopathy following massive transfusion. We shall consider the hemostatic disorders that are associated with MT, the degree to which staged transfusion regimens can prevent these problems, and what steps should be taken in the treatment of MVC.

Pathophysiology

The major primary event is a vascular lesion leading to blood loss and thus to the *loss* of hemostasis factors (including platelets). With a large wound surface area, the activation of hemostasis leads to a *consumption* of coagulation factors. The fluid shift causes a *dilution* of the hemostasis factors that remain within the vessels. The stress response mediated by vasopressin and epinephrine leads to an elevated level of specific hemostasis factors such as factor VIII (FVIII), von Willebrand factor (vWF), and tissue plasminogen activator (tPA). The process may be complicated by *disseminated intravascular coagulation* (DIC) triggered, for example, by the release of tissue thromboplastins from traumatized tissues. A major treatment priority is to establish an intravenous line for volume replacement, causing an increase in *dilution*. The use of plasma expanders can induce a further, specific hemostatic disturbance (e.g., the "coating" of platelets). The actual MT is not performed until the patient has reached the hospital, trauma unit, or operating suite and can further aggravate the preexisting, complex hemostatic disturbance. Efforts are made intra- and postoperatively to prevent MVB by means of appropriate replacement regimens (staged infusion of blood products) and, if necessary, to treat MVB with transfusions as directed by laboratory findings. We shall mainly consider diagnosis and treatment as they apply to multiple trauma victims.

Laboratory Findings

Lampl et al. [9] noted significant activation of plasmatic hemostasis, exceeding dilutional effects, at the accident scene in 20 multiple trauma patients. In particular, they found decreased levels of the inhibitors antithrombin III and protein C and increased levels of thrombin-antithrombin complexes. Fibrinolysis was also activated, as indicated by significantly elevated levels of tPA and fibrin(ogen) degradation products [10]. Kluft et al. [8] found extreme elevations of PAI-1 in 20 polytrauma patients 12 h after hospital admission. Seyfer et al. [14] compared hemostasis parameters in patients undergoing elective surgery and in patients with mild and severe multiple injuries. Significantly lowered levels of antithrombin III were noted intraoperatively in all patients with severe multiple trauma.

Boldt et al. [2] investigated hemostatic and platelet function in trauma patients. Platelet aggregation was found to be depressed in all patients, but platelet dysfunction did not normalize in the patients who developed sepsis. These differences were significant. Harrigan et al. [6] studied primary hemostasis in 22 injured patients who underwent massive transfusion (21 U of blood) and found that platelet function was depressed in all patients and that bleeding time was consistently prolonged. In more than 80% of cases the intra- and postoperative bleeding time was greater than 15 min, although no patients showed an abnormal bleeding diathesis. The authors concluded that the routine transfusion of platelet concentrates for the prevention of MVB is unwarranted.

Prophylaxis, Diagnosis, and Treatment

Staged transfusion regimens are used to minimize the extent of dilutional coagulopathy to ensure that any hemostatic disturbance will remain treatable and, if possible, to prevent bleeding in the massive transfusion setting. The regimens are varied, especially with regard to the initiation of FFP [1, 5], they were devised empirically, and they are not supported by controlled studies. Mannucci et al. [11] studied hemostasis and the efficacy of transfusion regimens in 172 patients who received an average of about 10 U of blood (RBCs or whole blood). They found no significant differences in terms of laboratory results and blood requirements among patients who received only RBCs or whole blood, patients who received RBCs and FFP, and patients who received RBCs, FFP and PC. They concluded that the routine prophylactic administration of FFP and PC had no positive effects in massively transfused patients. Reed et al. [12] performed a comparative prospective study to determine whether the routine administration of platelet concentrates would reduce the incidence of MVB compared with the administration of FFP. After receiving 12 U of modified whole blood or RBCs (the average transfusion was 20.6 U), each patient was given either 440 ml of PC or 440 ml of FFP. The incidence of MVB was equivalent in both groups: 18% and 19%, respectively. Again it was concluded that the routine administration of PC was not useful for reducing MVB. This study was later reevaluated to determine the ability of laboratory parameters to predict MVB [3]. In most cases thrombocytopenia was the leading cause of abnormal bleeding, followed by hypofibrinogenemia. The best predictors of bleeding were a fibrinogen level $\leq$0.5 g/l and a platelet count $\leq$50×10^9/l. Patients with fibrinogen and platelet values above these levels had only a 4% chance of developing MVB.

In the study by Counts et al. [4] in 27 trauma patients (with an average transfusion of 33 U per patient), eight patients developed abnormal bleeding, and in six of these patients bleeding was controlled with platelet concentrates alone.

References

1. Blauhut B, Lundsgard-Hansen P (1988) Akuter Blutverlust und Verbrennungen in der operativen Medizin. In: Mueller-Eckhardt (Hrsg) Transfusionsmedizin. Springer, Berlin Heidelberg New York, S 280–321
2. Boldt J, Menges T, Wollbrück M, Sonneborn S, Hempelmann G (1994) Platelet function in critically ill patients. Chest 106:899–903
3. Ciavarella D, Reed RL, Counts RB, Baron L, Pavlin E, Heimbach DM, Carrico CJ (1987) Clotting factor levels and the risk of diffuse microvascular bleeding in the massively transfused patient. Br J Haematol 67:365–368
4. Counts RB, Haisch C, Simon TL, Maxwell NG, Heimbach DM, Carrico CJ (1979) Hemostasis in massively transfused trauma patients. Ann Surg 190:91–99
5. Glück D, Kubanek B, Ahnefeld FW (1986) Die Therapie mit Blutkomponenten. Voraussetzungen, Indikationen und klinische Anwendung. Infusionsther 13:240–249
6. Harrigan C, Lucas CE, Ledgerwood AM, Walz DA, Mammen EF (1985) Serial changes in primary hemostasis after massive transfusion. Surgery 98:836–844
7. Hewitt PE, Machin SJ (1990) Massive blood transfusion. Br Med J 300:107–109
8. Kluft C, deBart ACW, Barthels M, Sturm J, Möller W (1988) Short-term extreme increases in plasminogen activator inhibitor 1 (PAI-1) in plasma of polytrauma patients. Fibrinolysis 2:223–226
9. Lampl L, Seifried E, Tisch M, Helm M, Maier B, Bock KH (1992a) Hämostasestörungen nach Polytrauma- Zum Verhalten physiologischer Gerinnunginhibitoren während der präklinischen Phase. Anästhesiol Intensivmed Notfallmed Schmerzther 27:31–36
10. Lampl L, Bock KH, Hartel W, Helm M, Tisch M, Seifried E (1992b) Hämostasestörungen nach Polytrauma- Zum Ausmaß der körpereigenen fibrinolytischen Aktivität während der präklinischen Phase. Chirurg 63:305–309
11. Mannucci PM, Federici AB, Sirchia G (1982) Hemostasis testing during massive blood replacement. A study of 172 cases. Vox Sang 42:113–123
12. Reed RL, Ciavarella D, Heimbach DM, Baron L, Pavlin E, Counts RBCJ (1986) Prophylactic platelet administration massive transfusion. Ann Surg 203:40–48
13. Sawyer PR, Harrison CR (1990) Massive transfusion in adults. Diagnoses, survival and Blood Bank support. Vox Sang 58:199–203
14. Seyfer AE, Seaber AV, Dombrose FA, Urbaniak JR (1981) Coagulation changes in elective surgery and trauma. Ann Surg 193:210–213

Subject Index